HEALING

SECRETS FOR ULTIMATE
FULFILLMENT IN LIFE

TIMOTHY J. SABO

Study Series

emerge
publishing

TULSA, OKLAHOMA

22 21 20 19 18 17   8 7 6 5 4 3 2 1

HEALING — 101 Things God Says About Your Health
©2017 Timothy J. Sabo

Published by:

TULSA, OKLAHOMA

Emerge Publishing, LLC
9521B Riverside Parkway, Suite 243
Tulsa, Oklahoma 74137
Phone: 888.407.4447
www.EmergePublishing.com

Author information contact:
Timothy J. Sabo Ministries, Inc.
5223 87 Street Edmonton, Alberta, Canada T6E 5L5
www.triumphantchurch.ca

Library of Congress Cataloging-in-Publication Data

ISBN: 978-1-943127-61-0 Paperback
ISBN: 978-1-943127-62-7 Digital/E-book

BISAC Category:
REL006680   RELIGION / Biblical Reference / Handbooks
HEA009000   HEALTH & FITNESS / Healing
MED034000   MEDICAL / Healing

Printed in the United States.

CONTENTS

INTRODUCTION

JESUS CHRIST STILL HEALS ALL

YOU HAVE BEEN DESTINED to live a *long* and *healthy* life! The last verse of Psalm 91:16 declares, **"With *long life* will I satisfy him, and shew him my salvation."** A long and healthy life is God's will for you! Jesus Christ bore all manner of sickness and disease when He was beaten, bloodied and bruised. Isaiah 53:4-5 and 1 Peter 2:24 both testify that by His stripes (the lashes Jesus received at the hand of Pontius Pilot) *you were healed.* Jesus paid the price for your healing.

In His earthly ministry **"Jesus went about all the cities and villages, teaching in their synagogues, and preaching the gospel of the kingdom, and *healing every sickness and disease among the people.*"** (Matthew 9:35) Hebrews 2:4 says that God confirmed the Gospel Jesus spoke about through the signs, wonders, and miracles He did. Many were brought to Jesus with demons, and He cast out the spirits with His Word and healed *all* that were sick.

Because Jesus is the healer of all, we can boldly declare His Word over our bodies:

"Let the weak say '*I am strong*!'"

"I *can* run through a troop and leap over a wall!"

"By my arms a bow of steel is broken!"

"I *can* do *all things* through the Anointed One and His Anointing which *strengthens me*!"

"I will *live* and *not die* and *declare the works of the Lord*!"

"I lay hands on the sick, and *they recover*!"

"God's Word is medicine to *all* my flesh."

"Jesus is the Lord that *healeth me*!"

CHAPTER ONE

HEALING IS GOD'S WILL FOR YOU!

LL THROUGHOUT THE WORD OF GOD we see examples of how Jesus confirmed God's promises and assured the sick that it was His will to heal them; there were none that He turned aside. Repeatedly the Word says, **"and he healed them all."** Take, for instance, the healing of the leper in Matthew 8. When the leper saw Jesus, he worshipped Him and said, **"Lord, if thou wilt, thou canst make me clean."** He wasn't really sure if Jesus would heal him. He probably knew Jesus *could* heal him (which is why he came to Jesus in the first place), but *would* he? Jesus immediately extinguished any doubts the leper had when He stated emphatically: *"I will; be thou clean."* With these two words, *"I will"*, Jesus cleared up any doubt concerning, not only this leper's healing, but our healing for today. After all, Jesus Christ is the same yesterday, today, and forever! (Hebrews 13:8) Just as Matthew 12:15 states, **"Great multitudes followed him, and *he healed them all,"*** Jesus still heals all today. Healing belongs to everyone who comes to Him; He will never turn anyone away. (John 6:37) Jesus did not just *say*, "It's My will," to the leper, but He *proved* His will by His actions.

Many a well-meaning Christian will say, "Well, if it be the Lord's will, I'll get better. If it be the Lord's will, I'll be healed." This may sound pious and humble, but it is in fact a great deception! God's Word declares in 2 Corinthians 1:20, **"For *all* the promises of God in him are *yea*, and in him *Amen*, unto the glory of God by us."**

Let's look at this verse closely: **"For *all* the promises,"** not just the one about salvation. *All* the promises! If you find a promise in the Word of God for your situation, guess what? It's yours!! We know that because the rest of this verse boldly declares, **"*All* of the promises are *yea*, and *Amen*."** God is not saying, "Hmm, I might heal that person. Maybe today I will deliver them from that affliction but maybe not." No! He is saying, "Yes! Amen! So be it! It's yours! Take it!" Sickness does not glorify God. What glorifies Him is when we walk in the manifestation of His promises: **"...unto the glory of God by us."** Healing brings God glory.

However, in order to walk in divine health, a decision has to be made to believe that it *is* God's will to heal your body. In actuality, healing is something that Jesus already *did*, past tense.

Look at this Scripture: **"By whose stripes ye *were* healed."** (1 Peter 2:24) The word *were* is in the past tense; it denotes something that has already happened. If **"ye *were* healed"**, then ye *are* healed! Every believer must settle their circumstance on the Word of God, knowing that it is absolutely God's plan and purpose for them to walk healthy all the days of their life! Then you will be able to boldly declare with the psalmist, **"I shall not die, but *live*, and declare the works of the LORD!"** (Psalm 118:17).

Consider this: Jesus said to the skeptical Pharisees who argued with Him about His right to forgive the sins of the paralytic, **"For whether is easier, to say, Thy sins be forgiven thee; or to say Arise, and walk?"** (Matthew 9:5) In essence, Jesus was declaring that the same Blood He would shed to save us from our sins is the same Blood that would heal our bodies. There is no difference. In fact, Isaiah 53:5 confirms this: **"But he was wounded for our transgressions, he was bruised for our iniquities: the chastisement of our peace was upon him; and with his stripes we are healed."** Salvation and healing were both purchased for us on the cross by the Blood of Jesus!

The Gospel of Jesus Christ is the **"power of God unto salvation to every one that believeth."** (Romans 1:16) Therefore, it is the quickening of our spirit, being made alive unto God our Father; it is the salvation of our soul, which is our mind, intellect, will and emotions; and it is healing and strength for our bodies. The word *salvation* in Romans 1:16 is translated *sōtēria* in the Greek and it means *deliverance, health, safety* and *salva-*

tion.[1]

Therefore we see that *salvation* means not only eternal life but the forgiveness of sins, healing, protection, provision, blessing, encouragement, and an infusion of the power of God, who is working in us, quickening our mortal bodies by His Spirit who dwells in us. (Romans 8:11) *That* is salvation. God sent His Word to heal us.

Today make a decision to believe that it is God's will to heal your body. Receive Jesus Christ (the Anointed One and His Anointing) as your Healer just like you have received Him as your Provider and Savior.

CHAPTER TWO

KNOW YOUR COVENANT RIGHTS

HEALING IS THE BREAD OF THE CHILDREN and it is our <u>Family Right</u>. When you ask Jesus into your heart and are born again, you become part of the Family of God and, as with a natural earthly family, children have certain rights and privileges. We can be confident that God, as our Father, has made provision through Jesus' sacrifice on the cross, for our complete healing: spirit, soul and body.

Healing is also our <u>Gospel Right</u>. The word *Gospel* in the Greek actually means *a good message* or *good news*[1] (news that seems almost too good to be true!), and that is exactly what healing is - Good News! God wrote a letter to humanity, and in it He shouted, "I have some Good News for you! My Son has purchased complete and total wholeness for your body, for your mind, for your emotions, for your relationships, for your marriage, for your finances! It is My will! I give you My Word on it!"

Healing is also our <u>Legal Right</u>. The New Testament is a legal document sealed by the Blood of Jesus. The word for *testament* in the Greek is *diathēkē,* which means a *contract* or a *covenant.*[2] Consider this: when a person passes away, they oftentimes leave an inheritance for their loved ones in the form of a will. We might call it their *last will and testament.* Jesus left us, in the form of the New Testament, a legal document stating God's will for us concerning our health and sealed it with His Blood. In fact, as He shared one last meal with His friends, He said, **"This is my blood of the new testament, which is shed for many."** (Mark 14:24) *The Living Bible* says it this way: **"This is my blood, poured out for many, sealing the new agreement between God and man."**

Healing is our <u>Redemptive Right</u>. As part of restoring the Blessing that He bestowed on Adam and Eve in the Garden of Eden long ago, God had a plan to redeem, or purchase back, every part of our spirit, soul, and body from the enemy. We call this God's *plan of redemption.* In Isaiah 53, we read that Jesus bore our griefs and sorrows, was wounded for our transgressions and crushed for our iniquities, that the chastisement for our peace was upon Him, and that by His stripes we were healed. God confirms His Word to us again in Matthew 8:17 when He says, **"He took our infirmities and bare our sicknesses"** and once more in 1 Peter 2:24, **" . . . by [His] stripes ye were healed."** Healing is definitely part of God's redemptive plan.

Healing is our <u>Needful Right</u>. God is a loving Father and a good Provider. Just as an earthly daddy takes care of the needs of his family and will do all that he can to provide for them, our heavenly Father has paved the way for restoration and completeness for us through the sacrifice of His Son on the cross. God saw that mankind was broken and sick, and He supplied them with wholeness and divine health. Healing is part of God's provision for His children.

Healing is our <u>Prayerful Right</u>. Whenever we ask for anything in accordance with God's will, we can be confident of the answer: **"For all the promises of God in Him are Yes, and in Him Amen, to the glory of God through us."** (2 Corinthians 1:20 NKJV) If you find a promise in the Word of God, you can take it and, as you take it, know that it gives God great glory when you receive it! Oftentimes people ask, "Is it God's will for me to be healed?" Be assured that God's *will* is His *Word*. He doesn't say one thing and will another. When He says something, He means it and will back it up. Settle it in your heart! Lester Sumrall used to say that to believe you receive your healing is to set a time and a moment, and say that, "From this time forward, I've got it!"

Know this: even Jesus Himself said, **"Whatever things you ask when you pray, believe that you receive them, and you will have them."** (Mark 11:24 NKJV) It is God's will for you to receive your healing when you pray.

CHAPTER THREE

REDEEMED FROM THE CURSE

THE CURSE OF THE LAW as recorded in Deuteronomy 28:15-68 lists the consequences for breaking God's commandments, with verse 61 summing up the curse as it pertains to your physical body: **"Also every sickness, and every plague, which is not written in the book of this law, them will the LORD bring upon thee, until thou be destroyed."**

However, Galatians 3:13-14,19 provides a wonderful promise: **"Christ hath *redeemed us* from the curse of the law, being made a curse for us: for it is written, Cursed is every one that hangeth on a tree: that the blessing of Abraham might come on the Gentiles through Jesus Christ; that we might receive the promise of the Spirit through faith. And if you are**

Christ's, then you are Abraham's seed, and heirs according to the promise." *That* is Good News! You are redeemed from every manner of sickness and disease! You have a covenant with God through the Blood of Jesus; now it is your responsibility to know your covenant-rights!

Let's study Deuteronomy 28:16-68 in the light of our redemption. You have been redeemed from:

Verse 16: "Cursed shalt thou be in the city, and cursed shalt thou be in the field." (or on your job)

Verse 17: "Cursed shall be thy basket and thy store." (i.e. wallet, income, dividends, and investments)

Verse 18: "Cursed shall be the fruit of thy body . . . (being unable to have children)

. . . the fruit of thy land . . . (assets not producing bumper crops or increasing in value)

. . . the increase of thy kine, and the flocks of thy sheep." (investments losing value instead of increasing; whatever you put your hand to not prospering like Deuteronomy 15:10 and 30:9 says it should; not doing the greater works that Jesus said we would do in John 14:12)

Verse 19: "Cursed shalt thou be when thou comest in, and cursed shalt thou be when thou goest out." (failure, nothing ever working out)

Verse 20: We are redeemed from " **. . . cursing, vexation, and rebuke, in all that thou settest thine hand unto for to do, until thou be destroyed, and until thou perish quickly; because of the wickedness of thy doings, whereby thou hast for-**

saken me." (being harassed, troubled, irritated, and frustrated)

Verse 21: We are redeemed from " . . . **the pestilence cleav(ing) unto thee, until [thou be] consumed from off the land whither thou goest to possess it.**" (i.e. disease after disease, contagious epidemics. Psalm 91 confirms that God is our Deliverer from pestilence, plague and all the attack of the enemy.)

Verse 22: We are redeemed from " . . . **[being struck with] consumption . . .** (Hebrew *shachepheth: emaciation*[1]*,* which is the state of being abnormally thin or weak, or a *wasting disease of the lungs*[1]. It can refer to tuberculosis, which is how it is rendered in *The Living Bible*[2], as well as cancer, diarrhea, malnutrition, kidney failure or malaria. It has also been translated *infectious diseases* in the *Good News Translation*[3].)

. . . and with a fever . . . (Hebrew *qaddachath: burning ague*[4]. It can refer to malaria or some other illness involving fever and shivering. It can also include extremely high fevers accompanied by headaches and, in severe circumstances, delirium.)

. . . and with an inflammation . . . (Hebrew *dalleqeth: burning fever* or *inflammation*[5]. It is translated *infection* by the *New English Translation*[6] and *growing pain* by the *New Life Version*[7].)

. . . and with an extreme burning . . . (severe fever; i.e. heat stroke and any sickness with fever such as influenza or erysipelas)

. . . and with the sword . . . (Many translations render this word as *drought* because in the original Hebrew it can mean *drought* or *a cutting instrument*[8].*)*

. . . and with blasting . . . (which is blight - an injury to crops caused by the dreaded east wind. With its scorching heat, this wind produced extensive damage to standing crops and vegetation. Its relationship to *mildew* could indicate a disease brought about by a fungus, the spores of which were carried by the wind. In modern vernacular, one could also associate damaged crops with a business that isn't prospering. We are redeemed from being affected by the curse in our lands and businesses because we are tithers and givers, and because of the Blessing of Abraham that is at work within our lives. [cf. Galatians 3:9; Malachi 3:10-12])

. . . and with mildew . . . (Hebrew *yeraqown: paleness* or a *greenish yellow* color[9]. It can infer jaundice whereby the skin turns a yellow color or can mean fungi-infected crops and vegetation.)

. . . and they shall pursue thee until thou perish." (imminent death)

Verses 23-26: "And thy heaven that is over thy head shall be brass, and the earth that is under thee shall be iron . . . the rain of thy land [shall be] powder and dust: from heaven shall it come down upon thee, until thou be destroyed. [Thou shalt be] smitten before thine enemies: thou shalt go out one way against them, and flee seven ways before them: and shalt be removed into all the kingdoms of the earth. And thy carcase shall be meat unto all fowls of the air, and unto the beasts of the earth, and no man shall fray them away." (job, investments, financial endeavors producing no increase, and assets not bringing in a yield; fleeing from the enemies that ran from you until, ultimately, your bodily presence, existence, and name are remembered no more)

Verse 27: "**[Thou will be smitten] with the botch of Egypt** . . . (Hebrew *shechiyn: inflammation, boils, ulcers,* or skin *eruptions*[10]. These could include psoriasis, eczema, and rosacea, as well as all diseases related to leprosy.)

. . . **and with the emerods** . . . (Hebrew *techor: a tumor*[11], especially those pertaining to the anus or colon, or hemorrhoids[11]. The *Knox Bible* translates *emerods* as a *swelling in the groin*[12].)

. . . **and with the scab** . . . (Hebrew *garab: scurvy*[13], which is a Vitamin C deficiency that causes swollen bleeding gums and loosening of teeth, and bleeding under the skin. The *New English Translation* has also interpreted *garab* as *eczema*[14].)

. . . **with the itch** . . . (anything that would cause you to scratch your skin including skin eruptions)

. . . **whereof thou canst not be healed.**"

Verse 28: "**[You will be smitten] with madness** . . . (*Madness* is also rendered *insanity* by the *Complete Jewish Bible*[15], *lose your mind* by the *Good News Translation*[16], *distracted* and *crazed in thy whits* by the *Knox Bible*[12] and *go crazy* by the *Common English Bible*[17]. In English usage, *madness* and its related terms *mad, madman* designate a number of human conditions, the most basic of which is unusual or bizarre behavior. *Madness* could include many forms of mental illness such as bipolarism, schizophrenia, and dementia, as well as impaired reasoning due to memory disorders.)

. . . **and blindness** . . . (lacking the ability to see)

. . . and astonishment of heart." (Hebrew *timmahown: consternation, bewilderment*[18] - feelings of anxiety or dismay, distress. The *New International Version* renders this phrase as *confusion of mind*[19], *Knox* translates it as *crazed in thy wits*[12], and *The Living Bible* calls it *fear and panic*[20].)

Verse 29: "And thou shalt grope at noonday, as the blind gropeth in darkness . . . (no direction in life)

. . . and thou shalt not prosper in thy ways: and thou shalt be only oppressed and spoiled evermore, and no man shall save thee." (everything working against you, everything failing, favor with no one)

Verses 30-31: "Thou shalt betroth a wife, and another man shall lie with her . . . (adultery and infidelity)

. . . thou shalt build an house, and thou shalt not dwell therein: thou shalt plant a vineyard, and shalt not gather the grapes thereof. Thine ox shall be slain before thine eyes, and thou shalt not eat thereof: thine ass shall be violently taken away from before thy face, and shall not be restored to thee: thy sheep shall be given unto thine enemies, and thou shalt have none to rescue them." (being in debt, seizure of property, foreclosure, bankruptcy, owing to others what you have worked hard for; not being able to enjoy the fruit of your labor)

Verse 32: "Thy sons and thy daughters shall be given unto another people, and thine eyes shall look, and fail with longing for them all the day long: and there shall be no might in thine hand." (raising your kids in the ways of God only to have the enemy steal their hearts while you stand by helplessly, unable to do anything about it; i.e. backslidden children)

Verse 33: "The fruit of thy land, and all thy labours, shall a nation which thou knowest not eat up; and thou shalt be only oppressed and crushed alway." (debt eating up all that you have worked so hard to gain)

Verse 34: "So that thou shalt be mad for the sight of thine eyes which thou shalt see." (frustration that all you have, your family, income, and assets, will be enjoyed by someone else)

Verse 35: "[You shall be smitten] in the knees, and in the legs, with a sore botch that cannot be healed, from the sole of thy foot unto the top of thy head." (Hebrew *shechiyn: inflammation, boils, ulcers,* or skin *eruptions*[10] - knee and leg problems resulting from boils, ulcers, or skin eruptions.)

Verse 36-40: "[Thou shalt be brought under subjection to] a nation which neither thou nor thy fathers have known; and there shalt thou serve other gods, wood and stone. And thou shalt become an astonishment, a proverb, and a byword, among all nations . . . Thou shalt carry much seed out into the field, and shalt gather but little in; for the locust shall consume it. Thou shalt plant vineyards, and dress them, but shalt neither drink of the wine, nor gather the grapes; for the worms shall eat them. Thou shalt have olive trees throughout all thy coasts, but thou shalt not anoint thyself with the oil; for thine olive shall cast his fruit." (paying big money for investments but getting only a little back; job bringing in little income and what is earned being consumed; more month than paycheck)

Verse 41: "Thou shalt beget sons and daughters, but thou shalt not enjoy them; for they shall go into captivity." (in the natural: kidnappings, molestations, losing custody; as well as losing their hearts, affection, loyalty, whereby they are influenced more by the world and their peers than you)

Verse 42: "All thy trees and fruit of thy land shall the locust consume." (debt and adverse circumstances consuming all your assets)

Verse 43: "The stranger that is within thee shall get up above thee very high; and thou shalt come down very low." (others receiving the promotion ahead of you; people that were "nobodies" becoming "somebodies" instead of you; demotion)

Verse 44: "He shall lend to thee, and thou shalt not lend to him: he shall be the head, and thou shalt be the tail." (being in debt and, as a result of this debt, being a slave to the banks and lending companies, unable to come out from underneath their thumb; financial burden and bondage)

Verse 45-52: "Moreover all these curses shall come upon thee, and shall pursue thee, and overtake thee, till thou be destroyed . . . they shall be upon thee for a sign and for a wonder, and upon thy seed for ever . . . thou [shalt] serve thine enemies . . . in hunger, and in thirst, and in nakedness, and in want of all things: and he shall put a yoke of iron upon thy neck, until he have destroyed thee. [A nation shall be brought against] thee from far, from the end of the earth, as swift as the eagle flieth; a nation whose tongue thou shalt not understand; a nation of fierce countenance, which

shall not regard the person of the old, nor shew favour to the young: and he shall eat the fruit of thy cattle, and the fruit of thy land, until thou be destroyed: which also shall not leave thee either corn, wine, or oil, or the increase of thy kine, or flocks of thy sheep, until he have destroyed thee. And he shall besiege thee in all thy gates, until thy high and fenced walls come down, wherein thou trustedst, throughout all thy land: and he shall besiege thee in all thy gates throughout all thy land, which the LORD thy God hath given thee." (being consumed in every area, eventually unto death; being in bondage with no way to escape; having all of your investments eaten up until you are brought to nothing; i.e. bankruptcy, foreclosure, law suits, etc.)

Verse 53-57: "And thou shalt eat the fruit of thine own body, the flesh of thy sons and of thy daughters, which the LORD thy God hath given thee, in the siege, and in the straitness, wherewith thine enemies shall distress thee: so that the man that is tender among you, and very delicate, his eye shall be evil toward his brother, and toward the wife of his bosom, and toward the remnant of his children which he shall leave: so that he will not give to any of them of the flesh of his children whom he shall eat: because he hath nothing left him in the siege, and in the straitness, wherewith thine enemies shall distress thee in all thy gates. The tender and delicate woman among you, which would not adventure to set the sole of her foot upon the ground for delicateness and tenderness, her eye shall be evil toward the husband of her bosom, and toward her son, and toward her daughter, and toward her young one that cometh out from between her feet, and toward her children which she shall bear: for she shall eat them for want of all things secretly in the siege and straitness, wherewith thine enemy shall distress thee in thy gates." (parents turning against their children, dealing with them harshly; husbands and wives, who were once tender toward each other and their children, becoming evil toward each other; i.e. strife and division within the family)

Verse 59: " . . . thy plagues [will be made] wonderful (extraordinary), and the plagues of thy seed, even great plagues, and of long continuance, and sore sicknesses, and of long continuance." (*Young's Literal Translation* renders *plagues* as *strokes*[21], whereas the *Good News Translation* calls them *incurable diseases and horrible epidemics*[22]. The *New American Standard Bible* translates this word as *severe and lasting plagues*[23], the *New American Bible* as *severe and constant calamities*[24], and the *Amplified* version as *extraordinary strokes and blows, great plagues of long continuance*[25] - i.e. cancers, long sicknesses that are protracted, hereditary illnesses, malignant or incurable diseases, obstinate problems, and severe long-lasting diseases)

Verse 61: "Also every sickness, and every plague, which is not written in the book of this law . . . will [be brought] upon thee, until thou be destroyed." (covering every possible sickness, ailment, or disease)

Verse 62: "And ye shall be left few in number, whereas ye were as the stars of heaven for multitude . . . " (decrease where there was once increase)

Verse 63-64: " . . . [ye will be brought] to nought; and ye shall be plucked from off the land whither thou goest to possess it. [. . . Ye shall be scattered] among all people, from the one end of the earth even unto the other; and there thou shalt serve other gods, which neither thou nor thy fathers have known, even wood and stone."** (i.e. eviction notices, foreclosures, decrease in populace until you are no more; no legacy)

Verse 65: "**And among these nations shalt thou find no ease, neither shall the sole of thy foot have rest . . .** (renting, leasing but never owning debt-free)

. . . [thou shalt have] a trembling heart, and failing of eyes, and sorrow of mind." (The *New International Version* translates *trembling heart . . . sorrow of mind* as an *anxious mind . . . a despairing heart*[26], and the *Common English Bible* renders it *agitated mind . . . depressed spirit*[27].)

Verse 66-67: "**And thy life shall hang in doubt before thee; and thou shalt fear day and night, and shalt have none assurance of thy life. In the morning thou shalt say, Would God it were even! and at even thou shalt say, Would God it were morning! for the fear of thine heart wherewith thou shalt fear, and for the sight of thine eyes which thou shalt see."** (fear of death and failure; no peace; constant worry and dread; never being content; constant agitation and unhappiness)

Verse 68: "**. . . [thou shalt be brought] into Egypt again . . . and there ye shall be sold unto your enemies for bondmen and bondwomen, and no man shall buy you."** (captivity where there was once deliverance, bondage where there was once freedom; no one will want to use your services or giftings)

*****

It is important when reading Deuteronomy 28:16-68 to read it in the light of our redemption. Every verse speaks of an area that Christ has redeemed you from; according to Galatians 3:13-14, Christ has redeemed you from the *entire* curse of the law!

Don't wait for a doctor's report about sickness! As soon as a symptom of the curse tries to come into your life in the form of sickness, debt, or lack, immediately take the following steps:

1. Go to the Lord and get His orders.
2. Get your eyes on the Word!
3. Read the Word out loud over your situation!
4. Then say, "I believe it! I take it. I thank you, Lord, for health and wholeness. I forgive if I have unforgiveness against anyone."

Take the medicine of the Word morning, noon, and night . . . as often as the Lord tells you! If others in your household experience symptoms of the curse, use this prescription on them too!

Here is a great way to confess the Word of God over any sickness or symptom: "According to Deuteronomy 28:61, (name the sickness trying to oppress you) is a part of the curse of the law, but according to Galatians 3:13-14, Christ Jesus has redeemed me from the curse of the law! Therefore, I no longer have (name the sickness), in Jesus name! According to God's Word, I am healed!" Whenever you may have anything in your body that does not line up to what the Word of God says about it, remember that you are the temple of the Holy Spirit! Continue to declare, "God is at work within (name that part of the body). Christ Jesus is the Healer of all!"

CHAPTER FOUR

TAKE YOUR MEDICINE!

OW CAN YOU KNOW BEYOND a shadow of a doubt that it is God's will to heal you? Herein lies the secret: **"Faith cometh by hearing, and hearing by the word of God."** (Romans 10:17) This is why the study of Jesus' life in healing, deliverance, and miracles is a must for every born again believer. Putting the Word of God before your eyes, in your ears, and in your mouth will cause your faith to grow in the area of healing. It will stop the "doubt-talk" and greatly increase the "faith-talk," causing your faith to grow as you hear yourself speak the Word!

"My people are destroyed for lack of knowledge." (Hosea 4:6) Many Christians today are perishing because they don't know the Word of God in the area of healing. By knowing the truth of what God says concerning your health, you can be set free from the work of the enemy, from his lies and deceptions.

"Ye shall know the truth, and the truth shall make you free." (John 8:32) The deception of the enemy is that Jesus doesn't heal all; He heals only as He wills which is not much of the time. But when we immerse ourselves in the truth of the Word of God, and we are diligent in it, that truth will set us free from the lies of Satan.

The very first step to victory in any area is to *put the Word of God first place.* Make a firm decision to put the Word of God in your ears and before your eyes day and night. You may say to yourself, "I don't have any time for the Word of God." Do you have time to sit in the doctor's office? Do you have time to lie in the hospital? You may say to yourself, "I'm too busy," but if you make a quality decision to turn off the television and computer, and lay aside those novels and newspapers, you will find that you actually have quite a bit of time to sow into the Word! Make a quality decision to change the channel on the TV to the holy men and women of God who are teaching, preaching, and ministering faith in God for your healing so that you get God's vision of divine health. Decide to sow to the Spirit so that you can reap life, instead of always sowing to the flesh and reaping corruption or death. (Galatians 6:8)

Here are some practical ways to put the Word first place:

1. Establish a daily Bible reading time and don't detract from it! You may need to schedule it into your day timer so that you stick with it! Be consistent.

2. Place Bibles or other good source materials in areas that

you can read them on your down-time; for instance, the coffee table, the kitchen table, your nightstand, the bathroom.

3. Have a notebook, pen, and sticky notes readily available while you read. Record any Scriptures you find regarding healing or the area you are believing God in. Post Scriptures on your bathroom mirror, by the kitchen sink, in your car, etc. for easy reference.

4. Arm yourself with good teaching on healing. There are some excellent ministries listed in Appendix Four that offer free podcasts and written material on healing. Have the Word of God regarding your circumstance playing as you get ready in the morning, in the car on the way to work, at nighttime before bed. Take notes, and study the principles being presented. Surround yourself with words of faith and healing; surround yourself also with others who are likeminded and in agreement with you.

5. Make a quality decision to lay aside materials that are not building or contributing to your faith. These may include novels, newspapers, magazines, television, social media, etc. Don't allow any of these things to squeeze out your time in the Word!

6. Meditate on the Scriptures you find regarding healing. The word *meditate* in the Hebrew is *hagah* and it literally means *to murmur, to ponder, to imagine, to study, to meditate, to mutter, to speak,* and *to utter*[1]. Think about what

the Word you are reading means to you at that moment, how you can apply it to your situation. Ask the Holy Spirit for wisdom and understanding regarding God's promises and how to lay hold of them.

7. Speak God's promises out loud. The confession of your mouth is a powerful tool! When we speak His Word, we have His guarantee that it will not return void. **"[My] word shall not return unto me void, but it shall accomplish that which I please, and it shall prosper in the thing whereto I sent it."** (Isaiah 55:11)

8. Call those things that be not as though they were. (Romans 4:17) In Genesis 1:2, when God looked out over our world and saw that the earth was covered with darkness and chaos, He never said, "Wow, it's sure dark out there!" No! He never stated what He saw with His "natural" eyes. Instead, our Father spoke what He *wanted* to see, and so He simply declared: "Light! Be!" Get out of the habit of speaking your illness over yourself. Get into the habit of speaking health and healing, for surely this is what you want to see happen!

9. Guard your tongue! **"Death and life are in the power of the tongue"** (Proverbs 18:21), in the words we choose to say. Your life is a ship and your tongue is the rudder, guiding your days into the harbor you are going. Let's choose life, and health, and healing, and wholeness with the words we speak! Refuse to speak anything that

is contrary to what you are believing God for. Ask the Holy Spirit for help: **"Set a guard, O LORD, over my mouth; keep watch over the door of my lips."** (Psalm 141:3 NKJV) As well, beware of filling your mouth with words of strife and division: **"Gentle words cause life and health; griping brings discouragement."** (Proverbs 15:4 TLB) Speaking words of death will only hinder the work of God in our lives.

10. Act on the Word of God! James writes that faith without works is dead. In fact, he says this two times! (James 2:20, 26) He also says, **"Shew me thy faith without thy works, and I will shew thee my faith by my works."** (James 2:18) As your faith is built up in the Word of God, start taking practical steps of faith as the Holy Spirit directs you. Move something that you couldn't move before, do something that you couldn't do before. Be a doer of the Word and not a hearer only. (James 1:22-25)

11. Praise God for the victory! Praise is the language of faith, and, according to Psalm 8:2, our praise stills the avenger. When we praise God and thank Him for His promises, we stop the work of the enemy in our lives!

Remember, the **"weapons of our warfare are not carnal, but mighty through God to the pulling down of strong holds."** (2 Corinthians 10:4) What are some strongholds that must be pulled down in the area of healing? Is it the traditions of men?

Bad reports? Wrong mindsets? Negative words spoken over us? Negative words that have come out of our own mouths? All of these strongholds can be pulled down by committing to remain in the Word, through prayer, both in our earthly and our heavenly language, through a right confession, and through praise.

CHAPTER FIVE

THE DOCTRINE OF THE LAYING ON OF HANDS

INASMUCH AS IT IS GOD'S WILL to heal you, it is His will that we carry on the ministry of Jesus here on the earth. In John 14:12, we read, **"He that believeth on me, the works that I do shall he do also; and greater works than these shall he do; because I go unto my Father."** What were the works of Jesus? 1 John 3:8 says, **"For this purpose the Son of God was manifested, that he might destroy the works of the devil,"** and that Jesus, **"went about doing good, and healing all that were oppressed of the devil; for God was with him."** (Acts 10:38) In what manner did Jesus heal the sick? In reading the Gospels, we see that two main ways are mentioned: speaking a word, as with the centurion's servant (Matthew 8:5-13), and the laying on of hands as when He touched Peter's mother so that the fever left her body. (Matthew 8:14-15)

So what about us as the Body of Christ today? What is our role concerning healing? Jesus made His will clear before He left this earth when He said, **"Go ye into all the world, and preach the gospel to every creature . . . and these signs shall follow them that believe; in my name shall they cast out devils; they shall speak with new tongues; they shall take up serpents; and if they drink any deadly thing, it shall not hurt them; they shall *lay hands on the sick, and they shall recover*."** (Mark 16:15, 17-18) Laying hands on the sick is one of the six fundamental principles of the doctrine of the Lord Jesus Christ listed in Hebrews 6:1-2. It is a sign that follows believers. Jesus Himself freely employed the laying on of hands to heal people.

Let's look at a couple of examples from the Gospels:

"And he could there do no mighty work, save that *he laid his hands upon a few sick folk*, and healed them." (Mark 6:5) It doesn't say that He *wouldn't* do mighty works, but that He *couldn't* because of their unbelief. However, the few that He did heal, in this instance, He healed by the laying on of hands.

"And he cometh to Bethsaida; and they bring a blind man unto him, and besought him to touch him. And he took the blind man by the hand, and led him out of the town; and when he had spit on his eyes, and put his hands upon him, he asked him if he saw ought. And he looked up, and said, I see men as trees, walking. After that he put his hands again upon his eyes, and made him look up: and he was restored, and saw every man clearly." (Mark 8:22-25) The blind man was healed when Jesus placed His hands on him, not once, but two times! It is scriptural to lay your hands on a sick person a second time, if need be.

"And, behold, there cometh one of the rulers of the synagogue, Jairus by name; and when he saw him, he fell at his feet, and besought him greatly, saying, My little daughter lieth at the point of death: I pray thee, come and *lay thy hands on her*, that she may be healed; and she shall live." (Mark 5:22-23) Jairus knew that if Jesus put His hands on his daughter, she would be made well. And that is exactly what happened! **"And he *took the damsel by the hand*, and said unto her, Talitha cumi; which is, being interpreted, Damsel, I say unto thee, arise."** (Mark 5:41) In other words, Jesus touched the little girl, and when He did she was completely restored!

Jesus laid hands on people who were sick, and He encouraged His disciples to do the same. In fact, He said that one of the signs that would follow those who believe is that, **"they shall lay hands on the sick, and they shall recover."** (Mark 16:18) As believers we have a responsibility to obey the Word of God, and here the Word of the Lord is to lay hands on the sick and see them recover. It is a sign to everyone that Jesus is alive and still working today. Unbelievers may argue that Jesus was just a man; they may worship Mohammed or Buddha or follow the ways of humanism, but it is very difficult to deny the power of God when someone receives their healing through the laying on of hands! The Great Commission is to preach the *whole* Gospel, not only the part about repentance or baptism but also the part about Jesus the Healer.

We can see that Jesus' disciples took Him seriously with re-gards to this doctrine: **"And *by the hands of the apostles* were many signs and wonders wrought among the people."** (Acts 5:12) The apostle Paul also practiced the laying on of hands, when he was shipwrecked on the island of Melita: **"And it came to pass, that the father of Publius lay sick of a fever and of a bloody flux: to whom Paul entered in, and prayed, and *laid his hands on him,* and healed him."** (Acts 28:8) The man was healed through the laying on of hands.

Some would try to explain away this doctrine and say that it passed away with the apostles and is not for us today, but this is a lie of the enemy! Jesus didn't say that these signs would follow only the apostles, but that these signs would follow the *believers*! That is you and I!! That is the entire Body of Christ! That is any-one who is a born-again believer! In the light of Hebrews 6:1-2, to say that the doctrine of the laying on of hands has passed away is to say that the doctrine of repentance or the doctrine of baptism has passed away; we can't pick and choose which fun-damental truth we want to keep! If the laying on of hands for healing has been done away with, no one would have a right to believe in the doctrine of repentance.

Christ's commission is still the same today for all who confess Him as their Lord. He still commands His Church in the same way He commanded the disciples: **"And as ye go, preach, say-ing, The kingdom of heaven is at hand. Heal the sick, cleanse the lepers, raise the dead, cast out devils: freely ye have re-**

ceived, freely give." (Matthew 10:7-8) He still commands us to, " . . . lay hands on the sick, and they shall recover." (Mark 16:18) Let's pray as the disciples did in the book of Acts when they said, "Now, Lord . . . enable your servants to speak your word with great boldness. Stretch out your hand to heal and perform signs and wonders through the name of your holy servant Jesus." (vs. 29-30, NIV) When is Christ stretching forth His hands to heal? He is doing it when we stretch forth our own hands, boldly laying them on the sick in Jesus' Name!

"But unto you that fear my name shall the Sun of righteousness arise with healing in his wings." (Malachi 4:2) Let's not take anything away from the doctrine of Jesus Christ. Let's choose to believe it all, reaching out our hands with His to heal the sick. In doing so, we will see signs, wonders, and miracles flow through us to restore health to others!

CHAPTER SIX

PRACTICAL MINISTRY FOR EVERY BELIEVER

THE DOCTRINE OF THE LAYING on of hands is a ministry for every believer in the Body of Christ, whether you are in the five-fold ministry or not. In these last days, God is calling on His whole family to pray for the sick so that He can be glorified in the earth, drawing many people unto Himself. Healing is a visible sign to all people that Jesus is alive! Included in this chapter is some everyday wisdom for those administering God's healing power to others:

1. BE LED BY THE HOLY SPIRIT.

"For as many as are led by the Spirit of God, they are the sons of God." (Romans 8:14)

"And it shall come to pass in that day, that his burden

shall be taken away from off thy shoulder, and his yoke from off thy neck, and the yoke shall be destroyed because of the anointing." (Isaiah 10:27)

"Then he answered and spake unto me, saying, This is the word of the LORD unto Zerubbabel, saying, Not by might, nor by power, but by my spirit, saith the LORD of hosts." (Zechariah 4:6)

2. PRAY IN FAITH.

"And the prayer of faith shall save the sick, and the Lord shall raise him up; and if he have committed sins, they shall be forgiven him. Confess your faults one to another, and pray one for another, that ye may be healed. The effectual fervent prayer of a righteous man availeth much." (James 5:15-16)

"(As it is written, I have made thee a father of many nations,) before him whom he believed, even God, who quickeneth the dead, and calleth those things which be not as though they were." (Romans 4:17)

Notice that Abraham, the "father of many nations," and God, our Heavenly Father, both called things that they didn't see into existence. They didn't speak what they saw with their natural eyes, but rather what they wanted to see happen. Don't be moved by what you see when you minister to others; instead be moved by the Word of God.

Speak to that mountain! Mark 11:22-23 says, **"And Jesus answering saith unto them, Have faith in God. For verily I say unto you, That whosoever shall *say* unto this mountain,**

Be thou removed, and be thou cast into the sea; and shall not doubt in his heart, but shall believe that those things which he *saith* shall come to pass; he shall have whatsoever he *saith*."

Faith in God talks back to the mountain facing it. It also commands the mountain where to go. Verse 24 directs us to, "... believe that ye receive ..." *before you physically see it,* "... and ye shall have ..." the thing you are believing God for. So we are to believe that the sick person we are praying for is raised up before we see it with our physical eyes.

Remember that Mark 16:17-18 says, **"And these signs shall follow them that believe; In my name shall they cast out devils; they shall speak with new tongues; They shall take up serpents; and if they drink any deadly thing, it shall not hurt them; they shall lay hands on the sick, and they shall recover."** We are protected as we minister to others. As we pray in the name of Jesus, we know that, **" ... at the name of Jesus every knee should bow, of things in heaven, and things in earth, and things under the earth; And that every tongue should confess that Jesus Christ is Lord, to the glory of God the Father."** (Philippians 2:10-11)

3. AFTER YOU HAVE DONE ALL, STAND!

"Put on the whole armour of God, that ye may be able to stand against the wiles of the devil. For we wrestle not against flesh and blood, but against principalities, against powers, against the rulers of the darkness of this world, against spir-

itual wickedness in high places. Wherefore take unto you the whole armour of God, that ye may be able to withstand in the evil day, and having done all, to stand. Stand therefore, having your loins girt about with truth, and having on the breastplate of righteousness; And your feet shod with the preparation of the gospel of peace; Above all, taking the shield of faith, wherewith ye shall be able to quench all the fiery darts of the wicked. And take the helmet of salvation, and the sword of the Spirit, which is the word of God: Praying always with all prayer and supplication in the Spirit, and watching thereunto with all perseverance and supplication for all saints." (Ephesians 6:11-18)

Our fight is a prayer fight to lay hold of all that God our Father says is ours. "Prayer-fruit" is the number one fruit we are to bear in this world: **"If ye abide in me, and my words abide in you, ye shall ask what ye will, and it shall be done unto you. Herein is my Father glorified, that ye bear much fruit; so shall ye be my disciples. Ye have not chosen me, but I have chosen you, and ordained you, that ye should go and bring forth fruit, and that your fruit should remain: that whatsoever ye shall ask of the Father in my name, he may give it you."** (John 15:7-8, 16)

4. REMEMBER THAT YOUR BLOOD COVENANT WITH GOD THE FATHER AND HIS SON INCLUDES HEALING.

In taking a last meal with His disciples, Jesus, in essence, said, "Take, eat. This is My body, shredded for your healing, imparting abundant life to you." (1 Corinthians 11:24-30) God declared in Leviticus 17:11 that the, **"life of all flesh is in the blood,"** and we know that the New Covenant of God's love toward us is sealed by the Blood of Jesus. Therefore we are "Blood-Blessed" by God the Father and His Son and Spirit. By Jesus Christ's stripes we were healed. (1Peter 2:24) When He bore those thirty-nine stripes, the Blood of Jesus came forth and washed our sicknesses and diseases away, bringing us the life of God. Divine health, wholeness, and healing were released to everyone who would believe and receive it. The Blood of Jesus is now continually flowing and working in us an eternal work of God's strength, bringing life wherever it flows!

5. REJOICE IN THE LORD ALWAYS!

"Rejoice in the Lord alway: and again I say, Rejoice." (Philippians 4:4)

Keep your peace and joy gauges on full as you minister God's healing power! Faith rejoices, gives thanks and is glad. Doubt despairs, complains and is sad.

6. NO "DOUBT TALK"; ONLY FAITH TALK.

"Death and life are in the power of the tongue . . ." (Proverbs 18:21) What are you saying about what you see before you? Exercise yourself unto Godliness (1Timothy 4:7): all things are possible with God; therefore every case is easy.

7. LEAVE THE ONE YOU ARE MINISTERING TO WITH NO REASON OR EXCUSE TO BE SICK ANOTHER MOMENT.

Encourage the person that you are praying for to receive God's healing anointing. All they have to do is simply say, "Thank you, Jesus! I receive!" and enter into the Blessing.

"**Therefore I say unto you, What things soever ye desire, when ye pray, believe that ye receive them, and ye shall have them.**" (Mark 11:24)

8. YOU ARE BLESSED.

"**Blessed be the God and Father of our Lord Jesus Christ, who hath blessed us with all spiritual blessings in heavenly places in Christ.**" (Ephesians 1:3)

"**Christ hath redeemed us from the curse of the law, being made a curse for us: for it is written, Cursed is every one that hangeth on a tree: that the blessing of Abraham might come on the Gentiles through Jesus Christ; that we might receive the promise of the Spirit through faith. And if ye be Christ's, then are ye Abraham's seed, and heirs according to the promise.**" (Galatians 3:13-14, 29)

CHAPTER SEVEN

THE GIFTS OF HEALING

"Now there are diversities of gifts, but the same Spirit.
For to one is given by the Spirit the word of wisdom;
to another the word of knowledge by the same Spirit;
to another faith by the same Spirit;
to another *the gifts of healing* by the same Spirit..."
(ICorinthians 12:4, 7-9)

O NE VERY STRONG CONFIRMING ACTION in Scripture, which has been revealed by the Trinity, declaring and showing us that it is God's will to heal all the sick, is what the Bible calls the *Gifts of Healing*. Notice that the word "gifts" is in the plural. I believe this is to show that, as many diseases as have ever existed, there are just as many Gifts of Healing to cure them all. Think of it this way: just as a cluster of grapes on a vine is not considered a single grape, but many, so it is with the Gifts of Healing. They are a special ministry for curing all sickness, pain, and oppression by the power and Word of God, even raising the dead to life.

As we read in 1 Corinthians 12:9, the Gifts of Healing are a manifestation of the Holy Spirit to minister healing to others. They are another way of receiving our healing and are operated "as the Spirit wills", not "as I will". 1 John 3:8 says that the Son of God was made manifest to "destroy the works of the devil," so we can conclude that the purpose of the Gifts of Healing is to destroy the works of the devil in the human body by delivering and healing the sick.

The Gifts of Healing have nothing to do with medical science or human learning because they are made manifest by the power of the Holy Spirit. In fact, it is the same Spirit who raised Christ from the dead that releases resurrection power towards those oppressed in their bodies, making them whole to the glory of God, and, thus, these gifts are given as the Spirit wills. 1 Corinthians 12:28 confirms this by saying, **"And God hath set some in the church, first apostles, secondarily prophets, thirdly teachers, after that miracles, then *gifts of healings*, helps, governments, diversities of tongues."** Jesus is the perfect example of this described in Acts 10:38: **"How God anointed Jesus of Nazareth with the Holy Ghost and with power: who went about doing good, and *healing all that were oppressed of the devil*; for God was with Him."** Christ Jesus was the Gifts of Healing personified, and they operated through Him by the Holy Spirit. Jesus Christ our Lord, the Head of the Church, has now given these administrations to His Body, which we are in Christ the

Anointed One. Hebrews 2:4 says that God bore them **"witness, both with signs and wonders, and with divers miracles, and the gifts of the Holy Ghost..."** Now, as Christ's Body, we are to **"desire spiritual gifts"** (1 Corinthians 4:1), **"covet earnestly the best gifts"** (1 Corinthians 12:31), and, being zealous of spiritual gifts, **"seek that ye may excel to the edifying of the church"** (1 Corinthians 14:12).

There are many examples of the Gifts of Healing operating in the New Testament. In fact, the Gifts of Healing are actually the predominant gift of the New Testament, whereas, in the Old Testament the gift of the Working of Miracles was predominant. Take Jesus for instance: He healed all that came to Him and gave an open invitation for all sick people to be healed. We also read about the apostle Peter, whom had handkerchiefs and aprons that touched his body taken from him and, upon whose bodies they were laid, they were healed. Furthermore, when they brought the sick out into the streets, just the passing of Peter's shadow upon them would heal them. Another example is that of Paul the apostle and Barnabas who silenced a whole multitude and made them give them audience as they declared the miracles and wonders God had wrought among the Gentiles by them. (Acts 15:12)

These Gifts of Healing have not passed away with the early Church as some have mistakenly assumed. John G. Lake was a modern day apostle who had hundreds of thousands of documented notable miracles of healing through his prayer rooms in Spokane, Washington.[1] Alexander Dowie was another leader who operated in the Gifts of Healing in Chicago where he lived, starting his own city of Zion, Illinois; many were healed that came there to be ministered to by him. There were also the great tent crusades run by men like Oral Roberts, A.A. Allen, R.W. Schambach; packed out meetings with the likes of Kathryn Kuhlman, Aimee Semple McPherson, and Smith Wigglesworth; not to mention the healing ministries of F.F. Bosworth, T.L. and Daisy Osborn, Charles and Francis Hunter . . . and the list goes on. All of these men and women were Gifts of Healing Christ gave us. Numerous others have Gifts of Healing operating in their ministry today by the Holy Spirit, and by this we see Hebrews 13:8 being fulfilled: **"Jesus Christ the same yesterday, and to day, and for ever."**

I personally knew of a man named Brother Lawson in Accra, Ghana, West Africa, around 1975 - 1989, who would preach Scripture after Scripture on healing. He would then stop and lay his hands on a tree and tell everyone who was sick in the audience to go and touch the tree, and they would all be healed. Also, at times, he would stop preaching and take off dancing in the Holy Ghost, and everyone in the audience that was sick would be healed.

Just like water comes in many forms: ice, snow, frost, steam, clouds, hail; yet, in the right temperature, all will flow as water, the Gifts of Healing we see working differently and uniquely in various ministers are manifestations of the same Healer, Jesus. 1 Corinthians 12:4 says, **"Now there are diversities of gifts, but the same Lord,"** and verse 6, **"And there are diversities** of operations, but it is the same God which worketh all in all." As well, "There are differences of administrations, but the same Lord." (1 Corinthians 12:5) And we cannot forget that it is God who "set some in the church, first apostles, secondarily prophets, thirdly teachers, after that miracles, then *gifts of healings*, helps, governments, diversities of tongues." (1 Corinthians 12:28)

In the Old Testament, we see Elijah telling the Syrian general to go wash in the muddy Jordan River, dipping seven times and being healed of leprosy. (2 Kings 5) Another time Isaiah tells Hezekiah to put a fig poultice or salve on the boils that he had, and he was healed. (Isaiah 38:1-8, 21) In the New Testament, Jesus spit in a blind man's eye one time, and the man received his sight. (Mark 8:22-25) Another instance tells of how Jesus told a different blind man to wash his eyes in the pool of Siloam (John 9:6-7); both men were healed, though the method varied. Peter's shadow healed the sick. (Acts 5:15) Handkerchiefs and aprons had the healing power of God transferred into them, and the sick were healed. (Acts 19:11-12)

We also see throughout history those having manifestations of the Gifts of Healing having very specific diseases healed through them. For example, Philip the Evangelist cast the devil out of many in Samaria, and "many taken with palsies, and that were lame, were healed." (Acts 8:7) Reverend Smith Wigglesworth was specifically drawn to people who had internal trouble, particularly people with appendicitis, colic, or some internal disorder and was very used by God in getting them healed. I've heard of a man named Stephen Jefferys who had a tremendous manifestation of the Gifts of Healing in getting arthritic people healed. Kenneth E. Hagin pointed out in his own ministry that ruptures, growths, hernias, or lumps of any kind were almost always healed when he prayed for people.

As mentioned in 1 Corinthians 12:5, **"There are differences of administrations, but the same Lord."** The "administrations" mentioned here are Gifts of Healing, believers equipped by Christ to bless others with the healing of specific ailments. (1 Corinthians 12:28) The Gifts of Healing manifestation by the Holy Spirit are oftentimes very specific to each individual minister. Many times Gifts of Healing by the Holy Spirit operate in Evangelists. 1 Cor. 12 at the beginning calls the Gift of the Holy Ghost, Gifts of Healing. At the end of 1 Cor. 12 we see an administration of Christ called Gifts of Healings. These are people who operate in Gifts of Healings very predominantly. A Evangelist has the Gift of The Holy Ghost operating in them often. Usually it is a very specific disease or few they predominantly get healed. The Gifts of Healings: administration of Christ has many different diseases cured under their ministry regularly.

Now a comment or issue needs to be addressed in order to help sick folks looking for their healing: in Galatians 3:2, 5 Paul talks about the Holy Spirit being brought on the scene and miracles being wrought by the **"hearing of faith."** Some people are waiting for a Holy Ghost manifestation of the Gifts of Healing; however, remember that the Gifts of Healing are as the Spirit wills. Reverend Kenneth E. Hagin told us often in school at

Rhema Bible Training Centre, "We minister to people with all the ability we have and with all God gives us, but we don't operate the gifts of the Spirit as *we* will; it is as *the Spirit* wills." If there are no Gifts of Healing in manifestation, people can always be healed and set free based on the Word of God. The Word of God is anointed and **"the yoke shall be destroyed because of the anointing."** (Isaiah 10:27)

The **"hearing of faith"** mentioned in Galatians 3, when preached or taught and received by the hearer, can activate the Gifts of Healing. For example, Acts 14:8-10 mentions the man at Lystra who heard Paul declare that it was God's will for him to be made whole. In hearing this Good News, the Word of God, he received the faith to be made whole. Notice that as believers we can activate and bring the desired healing from Heaven by our faith in God and His Word.

Once we have received the Word of God on our particular situation, we can **"hold fast the profession of our faith,"** and thereby receive our healing (Hebrews 10:23). Mark 11:22-24 tells us how faith in God speaks and acts. By first getting God's Word on your specific disease, you can then fill your mouth with that promise and declare it over your body. For example, 1 Peter 2:24 assures us, **"by whose stripes ye were healed."** Think about what this verse means to you in your situation, your illness, how Jesus' whippings guaranteed your healing. Now speak it over and over, "By His stripes, I was healed." Talking and speaking out loud while listening to your mouth say, "By Christ Jesus stripes I was healed," will give you faith to talk back to the sicknesses or disease and make the devil and his cohorts pack their bags and leave! Even James 5:13-15 tells us that if any are afflicted with sickness and disease they should pray the prayer of faith. Then, put action to your faith confession! Do something you couldn't do before; move your arm, get out of bed, wiggle your toes. Mark 11:24 tells us, **"What things soever ye desire, when ye pray, believe that ye receive them, and ye shall have them."**

We can have more manifestations of God in our midst if we remember that where two or three are gathered together in Jesus' Name, He is in our midst. Our faith in God will accomplish mighty things because Jesus Christ is alive. The Holy Spirit will manifest Himself in His powerful Gifts of Healings as we stay in faith, knowing that God's great love and mercy towards us is to see each of His children live in divine health and to satisfy us with long life. This is why it is important for believers to be part of a local church where the Word of God is preached, and where they are under the spout where the Glory of God is being poured out. It's a whole lot easier to receive whatever it is you need from God where the Spirit of God is moving and working rather than on your own, especially when you are surrounded with words of faith and love. The Body of Christ is the most powerful institution on the earth today and the gates of hell will not prevail against it.

The Holy Spirit is a gift from God. In order to have Him in the manifestation of the Gifts of Healing, there is a holy protocol that needs to be honored and kept. We are encouraged to desire, seek after, and, **"covet earnestly the best gifts,"** (1 Corinthians 12:31) in order to do the work that needs to be done. We are also encouraged to stir up the gift of God by spending time praying in the language of God supernaturally, the language of love, praying in other tongues (1 Corinthians 14:2; 1 Timothy 1:6). Jesus healed all the sick that came to Him, showing us the will of God our Father. He wants to continue to do so but it is by the Holy Spirit. One of the benefits of praying in other tongues is that the Holy Spirit, who raised Christ from the dead, will **"quicken your mortal bodies by his Spirit that dwelleth in you."** (Romans 8:11)

Truly, the more time we spend being filled with the Holy Spirit and staying filled with Him by giving thanks, rejoicing, and worshipping God our Father according to Ephesians 5:18-20, the stronger, wiser, healthier, richer, more knowledgeable we become. Then we will lay hold of all that is ours including divine health and wholeness, whether it is by our simple faith in God's Word, **"...by whose stripes ye were healed,"** (1Peter 2:24) or by the miraculous wonderful manifestations of the Gifts of Healing.

Live Long and Live Strong! Jesus Christ our Lord bore our sicknesses and diseases and whipped the devil in Hades so we can walk healed, live a long and blessed life, and dwell in divine health all the days of our life!

Glory and Hallelujah too!

CHAPTER EIGHT

101 THINGS GOD SAID ABOUT YOUR HEALTH

THE WORD OF GOD IS FULL of His promises concerning your health! Remember that His will is His Word. He will never say anything that He doesn't mean; after all, He is not a man that He should lie! (Numbers 23:19) As you read each one of these guarantees from God's Word on healing, hear the voice of the Holy Spirit. Read them out loud! Romans 10:17 says that faith comes by hearing, and hearing by the Word of God. As you speak these Scriptures aloud, your faith will grow in this area. Believe it! Receive it! Take it! God's divine health is yours today!

1. I am Lord that heals you. (Exodus 15:26)

2. Your days shall be one hundred and twenty years. (Genesis 6:3)

3. You shall be buried at a good old age. (Genesis 15:15)

4. You shall come to your grave at full age, as a sheaf of grain ripens in its season. (Job 5:26)

5. When I see the blood, I will pass over you, and the plague shall not be upon you to destroy you. (Exodus 12:13)

6. I will bless your food and your water, and I will take sickness away from the midst of you. (Exodus 23:25)

7. You will not suffer miscarriage or be barren. (Exodus 23:26*a*)

8. I will fulfill the number of your days. (Exodus 23:26*b*)

9. None of your men or women will be barren. (Deuteronomy 7:14)

10. I will not put any of the diseases you fear on you, but I will take all sickness away from you. (Deuteronomy 7:15)

11. It will be well with you, and your days shall be multiplied and prolonged as the days of heaven upon the earth. (Deuteronomy 11:9, 21)

12. I turned the curse into a blessing unto you, because I loved you. (Deuteronomy 23:5; Nehemiah 13:2)

13. I have redeemed you from every sickness and every plague. (Deuteronomy 28:61; Galatians 3:13)

14. I am your life and the length of your days. (Deuteronomy 30:20)

15. Your strength will last as long as you live. (Deuteronomy 33:25)

16. I have found a ransom for you; your flesh shall be fresher than a child's, and you shall return to the days of your youth. (Job 33:24, 25)

17. I have healed you and brought up your soul from the grave; I have kept you alive from going down into the pit. (Psalm 30:1, 2)

18. I will give you strength and bless you with peace. (Psalm 29:11)

19. I will preserve you and keep you alive. (Psalm 41:2)

20. I will strengthen you upon the bed of illness and sustain you on the sickbed. (Psalm 41:3)

21. I am the health of your countenance and your God. (Psalm 43:5)

22. No plague shall come near your dwelling. (Psalm 91:10)

23. I will satisfy you with long life. (Psalm 91:16)

24. I heal all your diseases. (Psalm 103:3)

25. I sent My Word and healed you and delivered you from your destructions. (Psalm 107:20)

26. You shall not die, but live, and declare the works of the Lord. (Psalm 118:17)

27. I heal your broken heart and bind up your wounds. (Psalm 147:3)

28. The years of your life shall be many. (Proverbs 4:10)

29. Trusting Me brings health to your flesh and strength to your bones. (Proverbs 3:8)

30. My Words are life to you, and health/medicine to all your flesh. (Proverbs 4:22)

31. (My) good report makes your bones healthy. (Proverbs 15:30)

32. (My) pleasant words are sweetness to your soul and health to your bones. (Proverbs 16:24)

33. My joy is your strength; a merry heart does good like medicine. (Nehemiah 8:10; Proverbs 17:22)

34. The eyes of the blind shall be opened and the ears of the deaf shall be unstopped. (Isaiah 35:5)

35. The tongue of the dumb shall sing. The tongue of the stammers shall be ready to speak plainly. (Isaiah 35:6; 32:4)

36. The lame man shall leap like a deer. (Isaiah 35:6)

37. I will recover you and make you to live. I am ready to save you. (Isaiah 38:16, 20)

38. I give power to the faint. I increase strength to them that have no might. (Isaiah 40:29)

39. I will renew your strength. I will strengthen and help you. (Isaiah 40:31; 41:10)

40. Even to your old age and gray hairs, I will carry you, and I will deliver you. (Isaiah 46:4)

41. I bore your sickness and I carried your pains. (Isaiah

53:4)

42. I was put to sickness for you. (Isaiah 53:10)

43. With My stripes you are healed. (Isaiah 53:5)

44. I will heal you. (Isaiah 57:19)

45. Your light shall break forth as the morning and your health shall spring forth speedily. (Isaiah 58:8)

46. I will restore health to you, and I will heal your wounds. (Jeremiah 30:17)

47. I will bring (you) health and healing, and I will cure you. (Jeremiah 33:6)

48. I will bind up that which was broken and will strengthen that which was sick. (Ezekiel 34:16)

49. I will cause breath to enter into you, and you shall live . . . and shall put My Spirit in you, and you shall live. (Ezekiel 37:5, 14)

50. Seek me and you shall live. (Amos 5:4, 6)

51. I have arisen with healing in My wings. (Malachi 4:2)

52. I am willing; be clean. (Matthew 8:3)

53. I took your infirmities; I bore your sicknesses. (Matthew 8:17)

54. If you're sick, you need a physician. I am the Lord, your Physician, who heals you. (Matthew 9:12; Exodus 15:26)

55. I am moved with compassion toward the sick, and I heal

them. (Matthew 14:14)

56. I heal all manner of sickness and all manner of disease. (Matthew 4:23)

57. According to your faith, be it unto you. (Matthew 9:29)

58. I give you power and authority over all unclean spirits to cast them out and to heal all manner of sickness and all manner of disease. (Matthew 10:1; Luke 9:1)

59. I healed them all, and I am the same yesterday, today, and forever. (Matthew 12:15; Luke 6:19; Hebrews 13:8)

60. As many as touch Me are made perfectly whole. (Matthew 14:36)

61. Healing is the children's bread. (Matthew 15:26)

62. I do all things well. I make the deaf to hear and the dumb to speak. (Mark 7:37)

63. If you can believe, all things are possible to him that believes. (Mark 9:23; 11:23, 24)

64. When hands are laid on you, you shall recover. (Mark 16:18)

65. My anointing heals the brokenhearted, and delivers the captives, recovers sight to the blind, and sets at liberty those that are bruised. (Luke 4:18; Isaiah 10:27; 61:1)

66. I heal all those who have need of healing. (Luke 9:11)

67. I have not come to destroy men's lives but to save them. (Luke 9:56)

68. I have given you authority over all the enemy's power;

nothing shall by any means hurt you. (Luke 10:19)

69. Sickness is a satanic bondage and you ought to be loosed from it today. (Luke 13:16; 2 Corinthians 6:2)

70. In Me is life. (John 1:4)

71. I am the bread of life; I give you life. (John 6:33, 35)

72. The words I speak to you are spirit and life. (John 6:63)

73. I have come that you might have life, and that you might have it more abundantly. (John 10:10)

74. I am the resurrection and the life. (John 11:25)

75. If you ask anything in My name, I will do it. (John 14:14)

76. Faith in My name makes you strong and gives you perfect soundness. (Acts 3:16)

77. I stretch forth My hand to heal. (Acts 4:30)

78. I, Jesus Christ, make you whole. (Acts 9:34)

79. I do good and heal all that are oppressed of the devil. (Acts 10:38)

80. My power causes diseases to depart from you. (Acts 19:12)

81. The law of the Spirit of life in Me has made you free from the law of sin and death. (Romans 8:2)

82. The same Spirit that raised Me from the dead now lives in you, and that Spirit quickens your mortal body. (Romans 8:11)

83. Your body is a member of Me. (1 Corinthians 6:15)

84. Your body is the temple of My Spirit, and you're to glorify Me in your body. (1 Corinthians 6:19, 20)

85. If you will rightly discern My body, which was broken for you, and judge yourself, you'll not be judged and you'll not be weak, sickly, or die prematurely. (1 Corinthians 11:29-31)

86. I have set gifts of healing in My body. (1 Corinthians 12:9)

87. My life will be made manifest in your mortal flesh. (2 Corinthians 4:10, 11)

88. I have delivered you from death, I do deliver you, and, if you trust Me, I will yet deliver you. (2 Corinthians 1:10)

89. I have given you My name and have put all things under your feet. (Ephesians 1:21, 22)

90. I want it to be well with you, and I want you to live long on the earth. (Ephesians 6:3)

91. I have delivered you from the power of darkness. (Colossians 1:13)

92. I will deliver you from every evil work and preserve you. (2 Timothy 4:18)

93. I tasted death for you. I destroyed the devil that had the power of death. I've delivered you from the fear of death and bondage. (Hebrews 2:9, 14, 15)

94. I wash your body with pure water. (Hebrews 10:22;

Ephesians 5:26)

95. Lift up the weak hands and the feeble knees. Don't let that which is lame be turned aside, but, rather, let Me heal it. (Hebrews 12:12-13)

96. Let the elders anoint you and pray the prayer of faith over you in My name, and I will raise you up. (James 5:14, 15)

97. Pray for one another, and I will heal you. (James 5:16)

98. By My stripes you were healed. (1 Peter 2:24)

99. My divine power has given to you all things that pertain unto life and godliness through the knowledge of Me. (2 Peter 1:3)

100. Whosoever desires, let him come and take of the water of life freely. (Revelation 22:17)

101. I wish above all things that you may be in health. (3 John2)

CHAPTER NINE

FAITH CONFESSIONS FOR DIVINE HEALTH

FATHER GOD, I THANK YOU that above all things I am prospering, and I am in health, even as my soul prospers. I am the seed of Abraham; my body is blessed, and my youth is renewed like the eagles'. You are Jehovah-Rapha and have taken sickness and disease away from the midst of me. My soul shall bless You, Lord, and forget not all Your benefits. You've forgiven all my iniquities, and You've healed all my diseases.

In the name of Jesus, I curse at the root every sickness, disease, pain, virus, and infirmity that has attacked my body or ever touches my body. I cast you out in Jesus' name! Devil, you get your lying symptoms out of here! Come out! You're illegal and have no authority in my life. My body is the holy temple of God and He is glorified by my total deliverance and healing.

I continue in God's Word, and because I know the truth, the truth has made me free. I am whole, of sound mind and body; an energized, revitalized, purified, exercised, transformed, renewed, restored, strengthened, power-packed power-house for God! I believe in the healing power of God to fill me, surround me, preserve me, and purify my entire system.

I am now in the Body of Christ and forever loosed from the bondage of infirmity. My health has sprung forth. There is no trace of sickness or disease in my body, and I will never be sick another day in my life, in Jesus' name.

I serve the Lord my God, and He blesses my bread and water and all my food and drink. If I eat or drink any deadly or harmful thing, it shall not hurt me. God has taken sickness away from the midst of me. Jesus was manifested to destroy the works of the devil, so every attack upon my health is destroyed. Jehovah-Shalom prevails over my body. He's healed every wound so that there's nothing missing, nothing broken. The Spirit of Him that raised up Jesus from the dead quickens my mortal body every day. I am dead to sins and alive unto righteousness. You healed me, O Lord, and I am healed in Jesus' name. Amen. Glory to God!

-Bill Winston: "Confession for Divine Health"[1]

*****

FATHER GOD, I THANK YOU I am Your child. I thank you for giving me the Name of Jesus and the authority that goes with it. Thank you for giving me Your Holy Spirit, the Greater One, the Mighty Power of God.

In Jesus' Name, I have authority over all demons, over all disease, to move obstacles, to stop problems, to calm storms, to rebuke sickness – I have authority! I have power! In Jesus' Name!

In Jesus' Name, fear and doubt leave me. Be gone. Confusion, deception, be gone. Heaviness, be gone. Depression, be gone in Jesus' Name. Mind, be strong, think clear, and be bright and sharp.

Soul, be strong. Have peace, be at rest and be free and loosed.

Body, be strong. Tumors and growths, anything that ought not be in the body, I speak against you. I command you in Jesus' Name to die, die, dry up, be gone and leave me!

I don't desire to eat so much that I become overweight. In Jesus' Name, I proclaim that my body is the temple of the Holy Ghost. Body, you settle down, and come into line with the Word of God in Jesus' Name. Be without spot, wrinkle, or blemish.

Heart, be clear. Be strong! Lungs, be clear. Be strong! Stomach, intestines, be healed. Be healed. Be whole. Be free. Work right! Every organ, every gland be right. Be normal. Be healthy. Be strong! Every bone, every muscle, every ligament, all my nerves, all my skin, be healthy. Be whole. Be right. Be strong in Jesus' Name.

Satan, in Jesus' Name I command you to take your hands off my money, off my finances, off my investments, off my business, off my job! In Jesus' Name, STOP in your operations and cease in your maneuvers!

Ministering spirits, angels, GO! Cause the money to come! Work, influence and cause it to come in Jesus' Name.

In Jesus' Name, Satan, stop in your operations against my marriage, against my family, and against my children! I forbid it! I bind you and you cannot continue. I stop it now in Jesus' Name!

My marriage is strong! My family is strong and free and right in Jesus' Name!

So be it!

-Keith Moore: "A Faith Confession"[2]

*****

GOD HAS DECLARED THAT HE would restore my health and heal me of every wound. I receive complete restoration, fresh flesh and vitality. There is nothing hopeless, for God has given me His Word that He would heal and cure the incurable. When others give up hope, I put my hope in God who gives me fresh flesh and complete healing!

- excerpt taken from "God's Healing Word" by Trina Hankins[3]

Appendix One

Healing: A Word Etymology

ONE EFFECTIVE WAY TO STUDY any given topic in the Bible is to do a word analysis. This is called *etymology* which, simply stated, means the explanation of where a word came from, or the history of a word.[1] For instance, the word *etymology* comes from the Greek word *etymon*, "true meaning of a word", and the Greek word *-logia*, "study, science".[2] Thus *etymology* is the science or study of the true meaning of a word!

In the *King James Version* of the Bible, there are six Hebrew words that are translated *healing* or *health* in the Old Testament and seven Greek words that are translated *heal (healing, healed, etc.)* in the New Testament. These words can be found by using the *Strong's Exhaustive Concordance*[3]. The Greek words can further be studied using such resources as the *Greek-English Lexicon of the New Testament* by Walter Bauer[4] or *The Analytical Lexicon to the Greek New Testament* by William D. Mounce.[5]

Below are listed each Hebrew word associated with the term *healing*, along with the *Strong's* reference number, how it is used in the *King James Bible*, and its definition:

rapha' (H7495): to mend (by stitching), i.e. (figuratively) to cure: -cure, (cause to) heal, physician, repair, make whole.

The KJV translates *rapha'* in the following manner: heal (57x), physician (5x), cure (1x), repaired (1x).

Therefore, *rapha'* means to heal, or make healthful.[6]

(Also see *riph'uwth* (H7500): a cure: -health.[7])

marpe' (H4832): curative, i.e. literally (concretely) a medicine, or (abstractly) a cure; (figuratively) deliverance: -healing, health, remedy, sound, wholesome.

The KJV translates *marpe'* in the following manner: health (5x), healing (3x), remedy (3x), cure (1x), sound (1x), wholesome (1x), yielding (1x).

Therefore, *marpe'* means health, healing, or cure.[8]

shalom (H7965): safe, i.e. (figuratively) well, happy; also (abstractly) welfare, i.e. health, prosperity, peace: -favor, (good) health, peace, prosper, prosperity, prosperous, rest, safe, safety, welfare, all is well, be well.

The KJV translates *shalom* in the following manner: peace

(175x), well (14x), peaceably (9x), welfare (5x), prosperity (4x), safe (3x), health (2x), peaceable (2x).

Therefore, shalom means completeness, soundness, welfare, and peace, even as it relates to one's health.[9] It means nothing missing, nothing broken - complete wholeness in every area of your life!

yeshua (H3444): something saved, i.e. (abstractly) deliverance; hence, aid, victory, prosperity: -deliverance, health, help (-ing), salvation, save, saving (health), welfare.

The KJV translates *yeshua* in the following manner: salvation (65x), help (4x), deliverance (3x), health (3x), save (1x), saving (1x), welfare (1x).

Therefore, *yeshua* means salvation, deliverance, wealth, prosperity and victory.[10]

'*arukah* (H724): restoring to soundness; wholeness; -health, made up, perfected.

The KJV translates '*arukah* in the following manner: health (4x), perfected (1x), made up (1x)

Therefore, '*arukah* means healing or restoration.[11]

Below are listed each Greek word associated with the word *healing*, along with the Strong's reference number, how it is used in the *King James Bible*, and its definition:

therapeuō (G2323): to wait upon menially, i.e. (figuratively) to adore (God), or (specially) to relieve (of disease): -cure, heal worship.

The KJV translates *therapeuō* in the following manner: heal (38x), cure (5x), and worship (1x).

Therefore, *therapeuō* means to heal, cure, or restore to health.[12] We get our English word *therapeutics* from this term.

iaomai (G2390): to cure (literally or figuratively); -heal, make whole.

The KJV translates *iaomai* in the following manner: heal (26x), make whole (2x).

Therefore, *iaomai* means to cure, heal, or make whole.[13]

Also see ***iama*** (G2386): a cure (the effect): -healing[14]; and ***iasis*** (G2392): curing (the act): -cure, heal, healing.[15]

sōzō (G4982): to save, i.e. deliver or protect (literally or figuratively): -heal, preserve, save, do well, be (make) whole.

The KJV translates *sōzō* in the following manner: save (93x), make whole (9x), heal (3x), be whole (2x).

Therefore, *sōzō* means to save; to keep safe and sound; to rescue from danger or destruction; to save a suffering one (from perishing), i.e. one suffering from disease; to make well, heal, or restore to health.[16] Simply stated, *sōzō* can be interpreted as healed and made whole.

Also see **diasōzō** (G1295): to save thoroughly, i.e. (by implication or analogy) to cure, preserve, rescue, etc.: -bring safe, escape (safe), heal, make perfectly whole, save.[17]

hygiainō (G5198): to have sound health, i.e. be well (in body): -be in health, be safe and sound, be whole.[18]

The KJV translates *hygiainō* in the following manner: sound (6x), be sound (1x), be whole (1x), whole (1x), wholesome (1x), be in health (1x), safe and sound (1x).[18]

Therefore, *hygiainō* means "to be sound, to be well, to be in good health"[18].

HEALING SCRIPTURES

"**Y**OU SHALL KNOW THE TRUTH **and the truth shall make you free.**" (John 8:32) These Scriptures are listed here that you may know the truth concerning your covenant-right on divine health and in knowing the truth that you would be made free! Begin today by looking up each one of these verses in your Bible; then, highlight or underline them, perhaps even write them in a notebook. As you do, let the Word of God sink deep into your spirit man. Read each Scripture aloud; meditate on each verse, asking the Holy Spirit to reveal a fuller understanding of them to you. Take the medicine of the Word, morning and evening, believing you receive each promise! His Word is His will for you!

Genesis 6:3	Psalm 29:11
Genesis 15:15	Psalm 30:1-3
Genesis 20:17	Psalm 34:19-20
Exodus 12:13	Psalm 41:2-3
Exodus 15:26	Psalm 42:11
Exodus 20:12	Psalm 43:5
Exodus 23:25-26	Psalm 67:2
Leviticus 26:9	Psalm 91:9-10
Numbers 23:19	Psalm 91:14-16
Deuteronomy 5:33	Psalm 103:1-5
Deuteronomy 7:14-15	Psalm 105:37
Deuteronomy 11:9, 21	Psalm 107:20
Deuteronomy 23:5	Psalm 118:17
Deuteronomy 28	Psalm 147:3
Deuteronomy 30:19-20	Proverbs 3:1-2
Deuteronomy 33:25	Proverbs 3:7-8
1 Kings 8:56	Proverbs 4:10
2 Kings 20:5	Proverbs 4:20-22
1 Chronicles 29:28	Proverbs 9:11
2 Chronicles 6:14	Proverbs 12:18
2 Chronicles 16:9	Proverbs 15:30
2 Chronicles 30:20	Proverbs 16:24
Nehemiah 8:10	Proverbs 17:22
Nehemiah 13:2	Isaiah 10:27
Job 5:26	Isaiah 35:4-6
Job 37:23	Isaiah 38:16, 20
Psalm 23:1	Isaiah 40:29-31

Isaiah 41:10

Isaiah 46:4

Isaiah 53:4-5

Isaiah 54:17

Isaiah 55:11-12

Isaiah 57:18-19

Isaiah 58:8

Isaiah 65:20, 22

Jeremiah 1:12

Jeremiah 17:14

Jeremiah 30:17

Jeremiah 33:6

Ezekiel 34:16

Ezekiel 37:5, 14

Hosea 13:14

Joel 3:10

Amos 5:4, 6

Nahum 1:9

Malachi 3:6

Malachi 4:2

Matthew 4:23-24

Matthew 6:9-10

Matthew 7:11

Matthew 8:2-3

Matthew 8: 5-9, 13

Matthew 8:14-17

Matthew 9:2-8

Matthew 9:18-26

Matthew 9:27-33

Matthew 9:35

Matthew 10:1

Matthew 11:5

Matthew 11:28-30

Matthew 12:9-13

Matthew 12:15

Matthew 12:22

Matthew 14:14

Matthew 14:35-36

Matthew 15:22-28

Matthew 15:30-31

Matthew 16:19

Matthew 17:14-18

Matthew 18:18-19

Matthew 19:2

Matthew 19:26

Matthew 20:29-34

Matthew 21:14

Matthew 21:21-22

Matthew 24:35

Mark 1:30-34

Mark 1:40-42

Mark 2:3-12

Mark 3:5

Mark 3:10

Mark 5:22-43

Mark 6:5

Mark 6:13

Mark 6:53-56

Mark 7:24-37

Mark 8:22-26

Mark 9:17-29

Mark 10:27

Mark 10:46-52

Mark 11:22-26

Mark 13:31

Mark 16:17-18

Luke 1:37-38, 45

Luke 4:16-21

Luke 4:38-41

Luke 5:12-13

Luke 5:17-26

Luke 6:6-10

Luke 6:17-19

Luke 7:2-10

Luke 7:12-15

Luke 7:21-22

Luke 8:2

Luke 8:41-55

Luke 9:1-2, 6

Luke 9:11

Luke 10:19

Luke 13:11-16

Luke 14:2-4

Luke 17:12-19

Luke 18:35-43

Luke 22:49-51

John 4:46-53

John 5:2-14

John 6:2

John 9:1-7

John 10:10

John 11:3-4, 43-44

John 12:1, 17-18

John 14:12-14

John 15:7

John 16:23-24

John 16:33

Acts 3:1-11, 16

Acts 4:22

Acts 4:30

Acts 5:12

Acts 5:15-16

Acts 6:8

Acts 8:6-7

Acts 9:33-35

Acts 9:36-41

Acts 10:38

Acts 14:3

Acts 14:8-10	1 Timothy 6:12
Acts 19:11-12	2 Timothy 1:7
Acts 20:9-12	Philemon 1:6
Acts 28:8-9	Hebrews 1:1-4
Romans 4:20	Hebrews 2:14-15
Romans 6:14	Hebrews 4:14-16
Romans 8:2	Hebrews 9:12
Romans 8:11	Hebrews 10:23
Romans 8:31-32	Hebrews 10:35-36
Romans 10:17	Hebrews 11:1
1 Corinthians 3:16	Hebrews 11:6
2 Corinthians 4:16-21	Hebrews 11:11
2 Corinthians 10:3-5	Hebrews 12:12-13
Galatians 3:13-14, 29	Hebrews 13:8
Ephesians 1:16-23	James 1:17
Ephesians 5:30	James 4:7
Ephesians 6:3	James 5:14-16
Ephesians 6:10-17	1 Peter 2:24
Philippians 1:6	1 John 3:8
Philippians 2:8-11	1 John 3:21-22
Philippians 4:6-9	1 John 4:4
Colossians 1:12-14	1 John 5:4-5
Colossians 2:10	1 John 5:14-15
Colossians 2:15	3 John 2
1 Thessalonians 5:23	Revelation 12:11

SPECIFIC SCRIPTURES FOR YOUR BODY

"**MY SON, ATTEND TO MY WORDS; incline thine ear unto my sayings. Let them not depart from thine eyes; keep them in the midst of thine heart. For they are life unto those that find them, and health to all their flesh.**" (Proverbs 4:20-22) God's Word is medicine! It is *life unto those that find them*. It is *health to all their flesh*. The key to your healing, to walking in divine health all the days of your life, to truly experience the victory of God in this area, is to take your medicine . . . every single day!

Whatever the enemy has attacked your body with, find the promise of God and meditate on it! Write it down, read it in different translations, study to show yourself approved, and receive what the Word has promised!

Abdomen

- Deuteronomy 28:27 . . . **"[Thou shalt be smitten] with the botch of Egypt . . .** (*botch:* H7822 *shechiyn* - inflammation; ulcer[1]) According to Galatians 3:13, Christ has redeemed us from the botch.

- Proverbs 3:8 . . . **It [God's law] shall be health to thy navel, and marrow to thy bones.**

- Proverbs 18:20 . . . **A man's belly shall be satisfied with the fruit of his mouth . . .**

- Acts 28:8 . . . **And it came to pass, that the father of Publius lay sick of a fever and of a bloody flux: to whom Paul entered in, and prayed, and laid his hands on him, and healed him.** (*bloody flux:* G1420 *dysenteria*-dysentery, bowel ailment[2])

See also: Digestion

Acne

- 2 Samuel 14:25 . . . **But in all Israel there was none to be so much praised as Absalom for his beauty: from the sole of his foot even to the crown of his head there was no blemish in him.** (Acts 10:34 says that God is no respecter of persons; if He did it for Absalom, He will do it for you.)

- Ephesians 5:27 . . . **That he might present it to himself a glorious church, not having spot, or wrinkle, or any** such thing; but that it should be holy and without blemish

- 1 Peter 1:18-19 . . . **Forasmuch as ye know that ye were not redeemed with corruptible things, as silver and gold, from your vain conversation received by the tradition from your fathers; but with the precious blood of Christ, as of a lamb without blemish and without spot.** (Genesis 1:27 says that we are created in His image; therefore, God's redemptive plan includes being without blemish and without spot.)

See also: Complexion/Flesh/Skin

Aids

See: Anemia/Blood/ Immune System

Allergies

- Genesis 1:29 . . . **And God said, Behold, I have given you every herb bearing seed, which is upon the face of all the earth, and every tree, in the which is the fruit of a tree yielding seed; to you it shall be for meat.**

- Genesis 9:3 . . . **Every moving thing that liveth shall be meat for you; even as the green herb have I given you all things.**

See also: Immune System/Respiratory System/Skin

Anemia

- Exodus 15:2 . . . The LORD is my strength and my song, and he has become my salvation . . .

- Psalm 27:1 . . . The LORD is my light and my salvation; whom shall I fear? The LORD is the strength of my life; of whom shall I be afraid?

- Isaiah 40:29, 31 . . . He giveth power to the faint; and to them that have no might he increaseth strength. They that wait upon the LORD shall renew their strength; they shall mount up with wings as eagles; they shall run, and not be weary; and they shall walk, and not faint.

See also: Blood

Ankles

See: Feet/Joints

Anorexia Nervosa

- Deuteronomy 28:22 . . . [Thou shalt be smitten] with a consumption . . . (consumption: H7829 shachepheth-emaciation which means an abnormal thinness caused by lack of nutrition or disease[3]) According to Galatians 3:13, Christ has redeemed us from emaciation.

See also: Eating Disorders

Aphasia
See: Speech Impediments and Disorders

Arthritis (Greek: "arthro"[4] — joint, "itis"[5] — inflammation.)

- Deuteronomy 28:22 . . . **[Thou shalt be smitten] with a consumption, and with a fever, and with an inflammation** . . . According to Galatians 3:13, Christ has redeemed us from inflammation.

- Mark 3:3-5 . . . **And he saith unto the man which had the withered hand, Stand forth. And he saith unto them, Is it lawful to do good on the sabbath days, or to do evil? to save life, or to kill? But they held their peace. And when he had looked round about on them with anger, being grieved for the hardness of their hearts, he saith unto the man, Stretch forth thine hand. And he stretched it out: and his hand was restored whole as the other.**

- Luke 13:11-13 . . . **And, behold, there was a woman which had a spirit of infirmity eighteen years, and was bowed together, and could in no wise lift up herself. And when Jesus saw her, he called her to him, and said unto her, Woman, thou art loosed from thine infirmity. And he laid his hands on her: and immediately she was made straight, and glorified God.**

See also: Bones, Specific part of the body

Asthma

See: Respiratory System/Skin

Back

- Psalm 145:14 . . . The LORD upholdeth all that fall, and raiseth up all those that be bowed down.

- Psalm 146:8 . . . The LORD openeth the eyes of the blind: the LORD raiseth them that are bowed down . . .

- Luke 13:11-13 . . . And behold, there was a woman which had a spirit of infirmity eighteen years, and was bowed together, and could in no wise lift up herself. And when Jesus saw her, he called her to him, and said unto her, Woman, thou art loosed from thine infirmity. And he laid his hands on her: and immediately she was made straight, and glorified God.

See also: Bones

Baldness

See: Hair

Barrenness

- Genesis 18:14 . . . Is any thing too hard for the LORD? At the time appointed I will return unto thee, according to the time of life, and Sarah shall have a son.

- Genesis 20:17 . . . **So Abraham prayed unto God: and God healed Abimelech, and his wife, and his maidservants; and they bare children.**

- Genesis 30:22 . . . **And God remembered Rachel, and God hearkened to her, and opened her womb.**

- Genesis 35:11 . . . **And God said unto him, I am God Almighty: be fruitful and multiply; a nation and a company of nations shall be of thee, and kings shall come out of thy loins.**

- Exodus 23:26 . . . **There shall nothing cast their young, nor be barren, in thy land: the number of thy days I will fulfil.**

- Leviticus 26:9 . . . **I will look favorably upon you, making you fertile and multiplying your people. And I will fulfill my covenant with you.** (NLT)

- Deuteronomy 7:13-15 . . . **And he will love thee, and bless thee, and multiply thee: he will also bless the fruit of thy womb, and the fruit of thy land . . . Thou shalt be blessed above all people: there shall not be male or female barren among you, or among your cattle. And the LORD will take away from thee all sickness, and will put none of the evil diseases of Egypt, which thou knowest, upon thee.**

- Psalm 113:9 . . . **He maketh the barren woman to keep house, and to be a joyful mother of children. Praise ye the LORD.**

- Psalm 127:3 ... **Lo, children are an heritage of the LORD: and the fruit of the womb is his reward.**

- Psalm 128:3 ... **Thy wife shall be as a fruitful vine by the sides of thine house: thy children like olive plants round about thy table.**

- Isaiah 54:1 ... **Sing, O barren, thou that didst not bear; break forth into singing, and cry aloud, thou that didst not travail with child: for more are the children of the desolate than the children of the married wife, saith the LORD.**

See also: Hereditary Diseases/Reproductive System

Blindness

- Matthew 15:30 ... **And great multitudes came unto him, having with them those that were lame, blind, dumb, maimed, and many others, and cast them down at Jesus' feet; and he healed them.**

- Luke 7:22 ... **Then Jesus answering said unto them, Go your way, and tell John what things ye have seen and heard; how that the blind see, the lame walk, the lepers are cleansed, the deaf hear, the dead are raised, to the poor the gospel is preached.**

See also: Eyes

Blood

- Ezekiel 16:6 ... **And when I passed by thee, and saw**

thee polluted in thine own blood, I said unto thee
when thou wast in thy blood, Live; yea, I said unto
thee when thou wast in thy blood, Live.

- Joel 3:21 . . . For I will cleanse their blood that I have
  not cleansed: for the LORD dwelleth in Zion.

- Mark 5:25-29 . . . And a certain woman, which had
  an issue of blood twelve years, and had suffered many
  things of many physicians, and had spent all that
  she had, and was nothing bettered, but rather grew
  worse, when she had heard of Jesus, came in the press
  behind, and touched his garment. For she said, If
  I may touch but his clothes, I shall be whole. And
  straightway the fountain of her blood was dried up;
  and she felt in her body that she was healed of that
  plague.

- (cf. Leviticus 17:11, 14; Proverbs 4:20-23)

See also: Bones/Immune System

Boils

See: Skin

Bones

- Psalm 34:20 . . . He keepeth all his bones: not one of
  them is broken.

- Psalm 35:10 . . . All my bones shall say, "LORD, who
  is like unto thee, which deliverest the poor from

him that is too strong for him, yea, the poor and the needy from him that spoileth him?

- Proverbs 3:8 . . . It [God's law] shall be health to thy navel, and marrow to thy bones.

- Proverbs 14:30 . . . A sound heart is the life of the flesh: but envy the rottenness of the bones.

- Proverbs 15:30 . . . The light of the eyes rejoiceth the heart: and a good report maketh the bones fat.

- Proverbs 17:22 . . . A merry heart doeth good like a medicine: but a broken spirit drieth the bones.

- Isaiah 58:11 . . . And the LORD will guide you continually, and satisfy your soul in drought, and strengthen your bones; you shall be like a watered garden, and like a spring of water, whose waters do not fail. (NKJV)

- Ezekiel 34:16 . . . [I] will bind up that which was broken, and will strengthen that which was sick . . .

- Ezekiel 37:3-5 . . . And He said to me, "Son of man, can these bones live?" So I answered, "O Lord GOD, You know." Again He said to me, "Prophesy to these bones, and say to them, 'O dry bones, hear the word of the LORD! Thus says the Lord GOD to these bones: "Surely I will cause breath to enter into you, and you shall live."'" (NKJV)

- Acts 3:6-7 . . . Then Peter said, Silver and gold have

I none; but such as I have give I thee: In the name
of Jesus Christ of Nazareth rise up and walk. And
he took him by the right hand, and lifted him up:
and immediately his feet and ankle bones received
strength.

- (cf. 2 Kings 13:21; Job 10:11-12; Psalm 51:8; Proverbs
  12:4; Jeremiah 20:9; Ezekiel 37:3-7; John 19:36)

Brain
See: Nervous System

Breast
See: Reproductive System

Breathing
- Genesis 2:7 . . . And the LORD God formed man of
  the dust of the ground, and breathed into his nostrils
  the breath of life; and man became a living soul.
- Isaiah 42:5 . . . Thus saith God the LORD, he that
  created the heavens, and stretched them out; he that
  spread forth the earth, and that which cometh out of
  it; he that giveth breath unto the people upon it, and
  spirit to them that walk therein.
- Ezekiel 37:5 . . . Thus saith the Lord GOD unto these
  bones; Behold, I will cause breath to enter into you,
  and ye shall live.

- Acts 17:25 . . . **Neither is worshipped with men's hands, as though he needed any thing, seeing he giveth to all life, and breath, and all things.**

See also: Nose/Respiratory System

Bronchitis

- Deuteronomy 28:61 . . . **Also every sickness, and every plague, which is not written in the book of this law, them will the LORD bring upon thee, until thou be destroyed.** According to Galatians 3:13, Christ has redeemed us from bronchitis as well as any other cough or cold symptoms.

See: Immune System/Respiratory System

Bulimia Nervosa

- Deuteronomy 28:22 . . . **[Thou shalt be smitten] with a consumption . . .** (*consumption:* H7829 *shachepheth*-emaciation which means an abnormal thinness caused by lack of nutrition or disease[3]) According to Galatians 3:13, Christ has redeemed us from emaciation.
- (cf: Psalm 34:8; 103:5)

See also: Eating Disorders

Burns

- Isaiah 43:2 . . . **When thou passest through the waters, I will be with thee; and through the rivers, they shall** not overflow thee: when thou walkest through the fire, thou shalt not be burned; neither shall the flame kindle upon thee.

- Daniel 3:27 . . . And the princes, governors, and captains, and the king's counsellors, being gathered together, saw these men, upon whose bodies the fire had no power, nor was an hair of their head singed, neither were their coats changed, nor the smell of fire had passed on them.

See also: Flesh/Skin

Cancer

- Deuteronomy 28:22, 27, 59, 61, 66-67 (See notes in Chapter Three: Redeemed from the Curse)

See also: Specific part of the body/Tumors

Cataracts

See: Eyes

Cerebral Palsy

- Philippians 4:13 . . . I can do all things through Christ which strengtheneth me.

See: Nervous System/Paralysis

Cholera

See: Diarrhea/Dysentery/ Immune System/Infection

Chronic Sickness

- Deuteronomy 28:59 . . . **Thy plagues [shall be] wonderful, and the plagues of thy seed, even great plagues, and of long continuance, and sore sicknesses, and of a long continuance.** According to Galatians 3:13, Christ has redeemed us from chronic sickness.

- Jeremiah 17:14 . . . **Heal me, O LORD, and I shall be healed; save me, and I will be saved: for thou art my praise.**

- Nahum 1:9 . . . **What do ye imagine against the LORD? he will make an utter end: affliction shall not rise up the second time.**

- 1 John 3:8 . . . **He that committeth sin is of the devil; for the devil sinneth from the beginning. For this purpose the Son of God was manifested, that he might destroy the works of the devil.**

Cold

- Deuteronomy 28:61 . . . **Also every sickness, and every plague, which is not written in the book of this law, them will the LORD bring upon thee, until thou be destroyed.** According to Galatians 3:13, Christ has redeemed us from cough and cold symptoms.

See: Immune System

Complexion

- Job 42:15 . . . And in all the land were no women found so fair as the daughters of Job: and their father gave them inheritance among their brethren.
- Ephesians 5:27 . . . That he might present it to himself a glorious church, not having spot, or wrinkle, or any such thing; but that it should be holy and without blemish.

Constipation

- Matthew 15:17 . . . Do not ye yet understand, that whatsoever entereth in at the mouth goeth into the belly, and is cast out into the draught?

Cuts

- Psalm 147:3 . . . He healeth the broken in heart, and bindeth up their wounds.
- Isaiah 53:5 . . . But he was wounded for our transgressions, he was bruised for our iniquities: the chastisement of our peace was upon him; and with his stripes we are healed.
- Jeremiah 30:17 . . . For I will restore health unto thee, and I will heal thee of thy wounds, saith the LORD . . .
- Ezekiel 34:16 . . . [I] will bind up that which was broken, and will strengthen that which was sick . . .

See also: Pain/Wounds

Cysts
See: Tumors

Dandruff
See: Hair/Itch /Skin

Deafness

* Matthew 15:30 . . . **And great multitudes came unto him, having with them those that were lame, blind, dumb, maimed, and many others, and cast them down at Jesus' feet; and he healed them.**

* Luke 7:22 . . . **Then Jesus answering said unto them, Go your way, and tell John what things ye have seen and heard; how that the blind see, the lame walk, the lepers are cleansed, the deaf hear, the dead are raised, to the poor the gospel is preached.**

See also: Ears

Depression

* Deuteronomy 28:65 . . . **And among these nations shalt thou find no ease, neither shall the sole of thy foot have rest: but [thou shalt have] there a trembling heart, and failing of eyes, and sorrow of mind.** (*New International Version* translates *trembling heart; sorrow of mind* as *an anxious mind; a despairing heart*, and the *Common English Bible* renders it *agitated mind; depressed*

spirit.) According to Galatians 3:13, Christ has redeemed us from depression.

- Nehemiah 8:10 . . . **The joy of the LORD is your
  strength.**

- Psalm 35:9 . . . **And my soul shall be joyful in the
  LORD: it shall rejoice in his salvation.**

- Proverbs 17:22 . . . **A merry heart doeth good like a
  medicine: but a broken spirit drieth the bones.**

- Isaiah 9:4 . . . **For thou hast broken the yoke of his
  burden, and the staff of his shoulder, the rod of his
  oppressor, as in the day of Midian.**

- Isaiah 10:27 . . . **And it shall come to pass in that
  day, that his burden shall be taken away from off thy
  shoulder, and his yoke from off thy neck, and the
  yoke shall be destroyed because of the anointing.**

- Isaiah 14:2 . . . **And the people shall take them, and
  bring them to their place: and the house of Israel
  shall possess them in the land of the LORD for the
  servants and handmaids: and they shall take them
  captives, whose captives they were; and they shall rule
  over their oppressors.**

- Isaiah 52:2 . . . **Shake thyself from the dust; arise, and
  sit down, O Jerusalem: loose thyself from the bands
  of thy neck, O captive daughter of Zion.**

- Isaiah 60:1 . . . **Arise [from the depression and pros-**

tration in which circumstances have kept you-rise to a new life]! Shine (be radiant with the glory of the Lord), for your light has come, and the glory of the Lord has risen upon you! (AMP)

- Isaiah 61:3 . . . To appoint unto them that mourn in Zion, to give unto them beauty for ashes, the oil of joy for mourning, the garment of praise for the spirit of heaviness; that they might be called trees of righteousness, the planting of the LORD, that he might be glorified.

- Philippians 4:4 . . . Rejoice in the Lord always: and again I say, Rejoice.

- James 4:7 . . . Submit yourselves therefore to God. Resist the devil, and he will flee from you.

- (cf. Psalm 147:3; Zechariah 9:8; Luke 10:19; 13:16)

See also: Mental Health/Nervousness/Oppression

Diabetes

- Deuteronomy 28:61 . . . Also every sickness, and every plague, which is not written in the book of this law . . . will [be brought] upon thee, until thou be destroyed. According to Galatians 3:13, Christ has redeemed us from diabetes.

- Proverbs 25:16 . . . Hast thou found honey? eat so much as is sufficient for thee, lest thou be filled therewith, and vomit it.

Diarrhea

- Acts 28:8 . . . **And it came to pass, that the father of Publius lay sick of a fever and of a bloody flux: to whom Paul entered in, and prayed, and laid his hands on him, and healed him.** (*bloody flux:* G1420 *dysenteria*-dysentery, bowel ailment[2])

See also: Abdomen/Digestion/Immune System /Poisoning

Digestion

- Psalm 22:26 . . . **The meek shall eat and be satisfied: they shall praise the LORD that seek him: your heart shall live for ever.**

- Ecclesiastes 3:13 . . . **And also that every man should eat and drink, and enjoy the good of all his labour, it is the gift of God.**

- Matthew 15:17 . . . **Do not ye yet understand, that whatsoever entereth in at the mouth goeth into the belly, and is cast out into the draught?**

- Mark 16:18 . . . **They shall take up serpents; and if they drink any deadly thing, it shall not hurt them. . .**

Discoid Lupus

See: Skin

Dysentery

See: Diarrhea

Ears

- Proverbs 20:12 . . . The hearing ear, and the seeing eye, the LORD hath made even both of them.

- Isaiah 29:18 . . . And in that day shall the deaf hear the words of the book, and the eyes of the blind shall see out of obscurity, and out of darkness.

- Isaiah 32:3 . . . And the eyes of them that see shall not be dim, and the ears of them that hear shall hearken.

- Isaiah 35:5 . . . Then the eyes of the blind shall be opened, and the ears of the deaf shall be unstopped.

- Isaiah 42:18 . . . Hear, ye deaf; and look, ye blind, that ye may see.

- Isaiah 50:4 . . . The Lord GOD hath given me the tongue of the learned, that I should know how to speak a word in season to him that is weary: he wakeneth morning by morning, he wakeneth mine ear to hear as the learned.

- Matthew 13:16 . . . But blessed are your eyes, for they see: and your ears, for they hear.

- (cf. Luke 22: 50-51)

Eating Disorders

- Daniel 1:15 . . . And at the end of ten days their countenances appeared fairer and fatter in flesh than all the children which did eat the portion of the king's meat.

- Ezekiel 37:6 . . . **And I will lay sinews upon you, and will bring up flesh upon you, and cover you with skin, and put breath in you, and ye shall live; and ye shall know that I am the LORD.**

See also: Abdomen/Digestion/Obesity

Eczema

- Deuteronomy 28:27... **[Thou shalt be smitten] with the botch of Egypt, and with the emerods, and with the scab, and with the itch** . . . According to Galatians 3:13, Christ has redeemed us from eczema.

See: Rash/Skin

Edema (also known as *dropsy*)

- Luke 14:2-4 . . . **And, behold, there was a certain man before him which had the dropsy. And Jesus answering spake unto the lawyers and Pharisees, saying, Is it lawful to heal on the sabbath day? And they held their peace. And he took him, and healed him, and let him go.**

See also: Feet/Legs

Epidemics

- Deuteronomy 28:22 . . . **[Thou shalt be smitten] with a consumption, and with a fever, and with an inflammation, and with an extreme burning, and with the**

sword, and with blasting, and with mildew; and they
shall pursue thee until thou perish. According to Galatians 3:13, Christ has redeemed us from epidemics.

- Psalm 91:3, 7, 10 . . . **Surely he shall deliver thee from
  the snare of the fowler, and from the noisome pestilence. A thousand shall fall at thy side, and ten thousand at thy right hand; but it shall not come nigh
  thee. There shall no evil befall thee, neither shall any
  plague come nigh thy dwelling.**

- (cf. Mark 16:18; Luke 10:19)

Epilepsy

- Matthew 4:24 . . . **So his fame spread throughout all
  Syria, and they brought him all the sick, those afflicted with various diseases and pains, those oppressed
  by demons, epileptics, and paralytics, and he healed
  them.** (ESV)

- Matthew 17:14-15, 18 . . . **And when they approached
  the multitude, a man came up to Him, kneeling
  before Him and saying, Lord, do pity and have mercy
  on my son, for he has epilepsy (is moonstruck) and
  he suffers terribly; for frequently he falls into the fire
  and many times into the water. Jesus rebuked the de-
  mon, and it came out of him, and the boy was cured
  instantly.** (AMP)

Eyes

- Deuteronomy 28:65 . . . **[Thou shalt have there] a trembling heart, and failing of eyes, and sorrow of mind.** According to Galatians 3:13, Christ has redeemed us from failing eyes.

- Deuteronomy 34:7 . . . **And Moses was an hundred and twenty years old when he died: his eye was not dim, nor his natural force abated.**

- Psalm 146:8 . . . **The LORD openeth the eyes of the blind: the LORD raiseth them that are bowed down . . .**

- Proverbs 20:12 . . . **The hearing ear, and the seeing eye, the LORD hath made even both of them.**

- Isaiah 29:18 . . . **And in that day shall the deaf hear the words of the book, and the eyes of the blind shall see out of obscurity, and out of darkness.**

- Isaiah 32:3 . . . **And the eyes of them that see shall not be dim, and the ears of them that hear shall hearken.**

- Isaiah 35:5 . . . **Then the eyes of the blind shall be opened, and the ears of the deaf shall be unstopped.**

- Matthew 13:16 . . . **But blessed are your eyes, for they see: and your ears, for they hear.**

- (cf. Leviticus 26:16; Deuteronomy 28:32, 65. According to Galatians 3:13, Christ has redeemed us from the curse of failing eyes.)

Fatigue

- Deuteronomy 34:7 . . . And Moses was an hundred and twenty years old when he died: his eye was not dim, nor his natural force abated.

- Psalm 18:32 . . . It is God that girdeth me with strength, and maketh my way perfect.

- Psalm 68:28, 35 . . . Thy God has commanded thy strength: strengthen, O God, that which thou hast wrought for us. The God of Israel is he that giveth strength and power unto his people.

- Joel 3:10 . . . Beat your plowshares into swords and your pruninghooks into spears: let the weak say, I am strong.

- Romans 8:11 . . . But if the Spirit of him that raised up Jesus from the dead dwell in you, he that raised up Christ from the dead shall also quicken your mortal bodies by his Spirit that dwelleth in you.

- 2 Corinthians 12:9-10 . . . And he saith unto me, My grace is sufficient for thee: for my strength is made perfect in weakness . . . for when I am weak, then am I strong.

- Ephesians: 6:10 . . . Finally, my brethren, be strong in the Lord, and in the power of his might.

- Philippians 4:13 . . . I can do all things through Christ which strengtheneth me.

- (cf. Nehemiah 8:10; Job 23:6; Psalm 27:1, 14; 28:7; 29:11; 71:16; 73:23-26; 84:4-7; 105:4; 138:3; Isaiah 26:4; 40:28-31; 41:10; Zechariah 10:12)

See also: Anemia

Fear

- Psalm 27:1 . . . **The LORD is my light and my salvation; whom shall I fear? The LORD is the strength of my life; of whom shall I be afraid?**
- Psalm 118:6 . . . **The LORD is on my side; I will not fear: what can man do unto me?**
- Isaiah 35:4 . . . **Say to them that are of a fearful heart, Be strong, fear not: behold, your God will come with vengeance, even God with a recompence; he will come and save you.**
- Isaiah 41:10 . . . **Fear thou not; for I am with thee: be not dismayed; for I am thy God: I will strengthen thee; yea, I will help thee; yea, I will uphold thee with the right hand of my righteousness.**
- Romans 8:15 . . . **For ye have not received the spirit of bondage again to fear; but ye have received the Spirit of adoption, whereby we cry, Abba, Father.**
- 2 Timothy 1:7 . . . **For God hath not given us the spirit of fear; but of power, and of love, and of a sound mind.**

- Hebrews 13:6 . . . **So that we may boldly say, The Lord is my helper, and I will not fear what man shall do unto me.**
- (cf. Psalm 118:6; Hebrews 2:14-15; 1 John 4:18)

Feet

- 1 Samuel 2:9 . . . **He will keep the feet of his saints . . .**
- Psalm 91:11-12 . . . **For he shall give his angels charge over thee, to keep thee in all thy ways. They shall bear thee up in their hands, lest thou dash thy foot against a stone.**
- Psalm 121:3 . . . **He will not suffer thy foot to be moved: he that keepeth thee will not slumber.**
- Proverbs 3:23, 26 . . . **Then shalt thou walk in thy way safely, and thy foot shall not stumble. For the LORD shall be thy confidence, and shall keep thy foot from being taken.**
- Song of Solomon 7:1 . . . **How beautiful are thy feet with shoes, O prince's daughter! the joints of thy thighs are like jewels, the work of the hands of a cunning workman.**
- Habakkuk 3:19 . . . **The LORD God is my strength, and he will make my feet like hinds' feet, and he will make me to walk upon mine high places.**
- Matthew 15:30 . . . **And great multitudes came unto**

him, having with them those that were lame, blind, dumb, maimed, and many others, and cast them down at Jesus' feet; and he healed them.

- Acts 3:7 . . . And he took him by the right hand, and lifted him up: and immediately his feet and ankle bones received strength.

- Acts 14:8-10 . . . And there sat a certain man at Lystra, impotent in his feet, being a cripple from his mother's womb, who never had walked: the same heard Paul speak: who stedfastly beholding him, and perceiving that he had faith to be healed, said with a loud voice, Stand upright on thy feet. And he leaped and walked.

- Romans 10:15 . . . And how shall they preach, except they be sent? as it is written, How beautiful are the feet of them that preach the gospel of peace, and bring glad tidings of good things!

- (cf. Deuteronomy 28:35 According to Galatians 3:13, Christ has redeemed us from foot problems; Psalm 22:16)

See also: Knees/Legs

Fever

- Deuteronomy 28:22 . . . [Thou shalt be smitten] with a consumption, and with a fever, and with an inflammation . . . (*inflammation:* H1816 *dalleqeth*-a burning fever[8]) According to Galatians 3:13, Christ has redeemed us from fever.

- Matthew 8:14-15 . . . **And when Jesus was come into Peter's house, he saw his wife's mother laid, and sick of a fever. And he touched her hand, and the fever left her: and she arose, and ministered unto them.**

- John 4:52 . . . **Then enquired he of them the hour when he began to amend. And they said unto him, Yesterday at the seventh hour the fever left him.**

- Acts 28:8 . . . **And it came to pass, that the father of Publius lay sick of a fever and of a bloody flux: to whom Paul entered in, and prayed, and laid his hands on him, and healed him.**

See also: Immune System

Flesh

- Job 33:25 . . . **His flesh shall be fresher than a child's: he shall return to the days of his youth.**

- Proverbs 3:8 . . . **It [God's law] will be health to your flesh, and strength to your bones.** (NKJV)

- Proverbs 4:20-22 . . . **My son, attend to my words; incline thine ear unto my sayings. Let them not depart from thine eyes; keep them in the midst of thine heart. For they are life unto those that find them, and health to all their flesh.**

- Ezekiel 37:6 . . . **And I will lay sinews upon you, and will bring up flesh upon you, and cover you with skin, and ye shall live . . .**
- Daniel 1:15 . . . **And at the end of ten days their countenances appeared fairer and fatter in flesh than all the children which did eat the portion of the king's meat.**
- 2 Corinthians 4:11 . . . **That the life also of Jesus might be made manifest in our mortal flesh . . .**
- (cf. Jeremiah 32:27; Luke 22:50-51; 24:39; Ephesians 5:28-32)

Flesh Eating Disease
See: Flesh/Necrotizing Fasciitis

Flu
See: Immune System

Glaucoma
See: Eyes

Groin

- Leviticus 21:18-21 . . . **For whatsoever man he be that hath a blemish, he shall not approach: a blind man, or a lame, or he that hath a flat nose, or any thing superfluous, or a man that is brokenfooted, or bro-**

kenhanded, or crookbackt, or a dwarf, or that hath a
blemish in his eye, or be scurvy, or scabbed, or hath
his stones broken; no man that hath a blemish of the
seed of Aaron the priest shall come nigh to offer the
offerings of the LORD made by fire: he hath a blemish; he shall not come nigh to offer the bread of his
God. (However, Revelation 1:6 states that God "hath
made us kings and priests unto God and his Father,"
and because we are priests, we are truly healed of these
things.)

- Deuteronomy 28:27 . . . [Thou shalt be smitten] with
  the botch of Egypt, and with the emerods . . . (emerods: H2914 *techor-* tumors, especially those pertaining
  to the anus or colon, or hemorrhoids[9]; the *Knox Bible*
  translates *emerods* as a *swelling in the groin*[10]. According
  to Galatians 3:13, Christ has redeemed us from all of
  these.)

- Proverbs 31:17 . . . She girdeth her loins with strength,
  and strengtheneth her arms.

- (cf. Ephesians 6:14)

Gums
See: Mouth

Hair
- Judges 16:22 . . . Howbeit the hair of his head began

to grow again after he was shaven.

- 2 Samuel 14:11 . . . And he said, As the LORD liveth, there shall not one hair of thy son fall to the earth.
- 2 Samuel 14:26 . . . He weighed the hair of his head at two hundred shekels after the king's weight.
- Proverbs 16:31 . . . The hoary head is a crown of glory, if it be found in the way of righteousness.
- Proverbs 20:29 . . . The glory of young men is their strength: and the beauty of old men is the grey head.
- Luke 12:7 . . . But even the very hairs of your head are all numbered . . .
- Luke 21:18 . . . But there shall not an hair of your head perish.
- (cf. 1 Samuel 14:45; 1 Kings 1:52; Psalm 103:5; Song of Solomon 4:1; 6:5; 7:5; Isaiah 46:4; Ezekiel 16:7; Daniel 3:27; Matthew 10:30; Acts 27:34; 1 Corinthians 11:15)

Hands

- Deuteronomy 33:7 . . . And this is the blessing of Judah . . . let his hands be sufficient for him . . .
- Nehemiah 6:9 . . . For they all made us afraid, saying, Their hands shall be weakened from the work, that it be not done. Now therefore, O God, strengthen my hands.

- Job 4:3 . . . Behold, thou hast instructed many, and thou hast strengthened the weak hands.
- Psalm 144:1 . . . Blessed be the LORD my strength which teacheth my hands to war, and my fingers to fight.
- Isaiah 35:3 . . . Strengthen ye the weak hands, and confirm the feeble knees.
- Mark 3:3-5 . . . And he saith unto the man which had the withered hand, Stand forth. And he saith unto them, Is it lawful to do good on the sabbath days, or to do evil? to save life, or to kill? But they held their peace. And when he had looked round about on them with anger, being grieved for the hardness of their hearts, he saith unto the man, Stretch forth thine hand. And he stretched it out: and his hand was restored whole as the other.
- Acts 4:30 . . . By stretching forth thine hand to heal; and that signs and wonders may be done by the name of thy holy child Jesus.
- Mark 16:18 . . . They shall take up serpents; and if they drink any deadly thing, it shall not hurt them; they shall lay hands on the sick, and they shall recover.
- (cf. Isaiah 41:13; Hosea 7:15)

Headache

- Psalm 103:4 **. . . Who redeemeth thy life from destruction; who crowneth thee with lovingkindness and tender mercies.**

- Isaiah 53:4 **. . . Surely He has borne our griefs (sicknesses, weaknesses, and distresses) and carried our sorrows and pains [of punishment]** . . . (AMP)

- 1 Corinthians 2:16 **. . . For who hath known the mind of the Lord, that he may instruct him? But we have the mind of Christ.** When you hear and believe a lie it causes bad feelings. But when you hear and believe the truth of God's Word it causes good feelings. Satan is the father of lies; so if he is trying to put a headache on you, don't believe the lie. Boldly declare aloud instead: "Satan and all of your cohorts, I rebuke you in the Name of Jesus, and I command you to cease in your operations. Stop in your maneuverings concerning my thinking process and imaginations. Thank you, Father God, for the mind of Christ. You have crowned me with loving-kindness and tender mercies. I receive the Word of God that restores my soul and renews my mind in Christ Jesus' Name.

- (cf. Matthew 16:19, 18:18; Luke 4:36, 9:1, 10:19)

Heart

- Deuteronomy 28:65 **. . . [Thou shalt have there] a**

trembling heart, and failing of eyes, and sorrow of mind. According to Galatians 3:13, Christ has redeemed us from a diseased or trembling heart.

- Psalm 22:26 . . . **The meek shall eat and be satisfied: they shall praise the LORD that seek him: your heart shall live for ever.**

- Psalm 27:14 . . . **Wait on the LORD: be of good courage, and he shall strengthen thine heart: wait, I say, on the LORD.**

- Psalm 73:26 . . . **My flesh and my heart faileth: but God is the strength of my heart, and my portion for ever.**

- Psalm 147:3 . . . **He healeth the broken in heart, and bindeth up their wounds.**

- Proverbs 14:30 . . . **A sound heart is the life of the flesh: but envy the rottenness of the bones.**

See also: Blood

Hemophilia

See: Blood/Hereditary Diseases

Hemorrhoids

- Deuteronomy 28:27 . . . **[You will be smitten] with the botch of Egypt, and with the emerods, and with the scab, and with the itch** . . . (*emerods:* H2914 *techor*-tumors, hemorrhoids, piles[9]) According to Galatians 3:13,

Christ has redeemed us from hemorrhoids.

Hepatitis
See: Immune System/Jaundice

Hereditary Diseases
* Deuteronomy 28:4 . . . **Blessed shall be the fruit of thy body.**
* (cf. Ezekiel 18:2-3; 20-21)

Hernia
See: Abdomen/Groin

Hips
See also: Arthritis/Knees/Legs

Hormones
See: Reproductive System

Immune System
* Exodus 11:7 . . . **The LORD doth put a difference between the Egyptians and Israel.**
* Deuteronomy 28:21 . . . **The pestilence [shall] cleave unto thee, until [thou be] consumed from off the land whither thou goest to possess it.** (*pestilence:* H1698 *deber*-pestilence, plague[11]*)* According to Gala-

tians 3:13, Christ has redeemed us from all manner of pestilence or plague.

- Psalm 3:3 . . . **But thou, O LORD, art a shield for me; my glory, and the lifter up of mine head.**
- Psalm 91:3, 7, 10 . . . **Surely he shall deliver thee from the snare of the fowler, and from the noisome pestilence. A thousand shall fall at thy side, and ten thousand at thy right hand; but it shall not come nigh thee. There shall no evil befall thee, neither shall any plague come nigh thy dwelling.**
- Proverbs 30:5 . . . **Every word of God is pure: he is a shield unto them that put their trust in him.**
- Isaiah 4:5 . . . **The LORD will create upon every dwelling place of mount Zion, and upon her assemblies, a cloud and smoke by day, and the shining of a flaming fire by night: for upon all the glory shall be a defence.**
- Romans 8:11 . . . **But if the Spirit of him that raised up Jesus from the dead dwell in you, he that raised up Christ from the dead shall also quicken your mortal bodies by his Spirit that dwelleth in you.**
- (cf. 1 John 4:4)

See also: Blood/Poisoning

Infection

See: Immune System

Influenza

See: Immune System

Insomnia

See: Sleep Disorders

Itch

- Deuteronomy 28:27 . . . **[Thou shalt be smitten] with the botch of Egypt, and with the emerods, and with the scab, and with the itch** . . . According to Galatians 3:13, Christ has redeemed us from anything associated with an itch.

Jaundice

- Deuteronomy 28:22 . . . **[Thou shalt be smitten with] a consumption, and with a fever, and with an inflammation, and with an extreme burning, and with the sword, and with blasting, and with mildew** . . . (*mildew:* H3420 *yeraqown*-paleness; greenish, yellow[12]. It can infer jaundice whereby the skin turns a yellow color.) According to Galatians 3:13, Christ has redeemed us from jaundice.

Jaw

- Hosea 11:4 . . . **I drew them with cords of a man, with bands of love: and I was to them as they that take off**

the yoke on their jaws, and I laid meat unto them.
See also: Mouth

Joints

- Song of Solomon 7:1 . . . **How beautiful are thy feet with shoes, O prince's daughter! the joints of thy thighs are like jewels, the work of the hands of a cunning workman.**
See: Arthritis/Specific part of the body

Keratitis

See: Eye

Kidneys

- Deuteronomy 28:61 . . . **Also every sickness, and every plague, which is not written in the book of this law . . . will [be brought] upon thee, until thou be destroyed.** According to Galatians 3:13, Christ has redeemed us from kidney stones/kidney infection/kidney failure.
See also: Infection

Knees

- Deuteronomy 28:35 . . . **[Thou shalt be smitten] in the knees, and in the legs, and with a sore botch that cannot be healed, from the sole of thy foot unto the**

top of thy head. According to Galatians 3:13, Christ has redeemed us from knee problems.

- Job 4:4 . . . **Thy words have upholden him that was falling, and thou hast strengthened the feeble knees.**

- Isaiah 35:3 . . . **Strengthen ye the weak hands, and confirm the feeble knees.**

- Hebrews 12:12 . . . **Wherefore lift up the hands which hang down, and the feeble knees.**

- (cf. Song of Solomon 7:1)

See also: Legs

Lameness

See: Feet/Hips/Knees/Legs/Paralysis

Learning Disabilities

- Psalm 119:99-100 . . . **I have more understanding than all my teachers: for thy testimonies are my meditation. I understand more than the ancients, because I keep thy precepts.**

- Isaiah 11:2-3 . . . **And the spirit of the LORD shall rest upon him, the spirit of wisdom and understanding, the spirit of counsel and might, the spirit of knowledge and of the fear of the LORD; and shall make him of quick understanding in the fear of the LORD . . .**

- Isaiah 54:13 . . . **And all thy children shall be taught of the LORD; and great shall be the peace of thy children.**

- Daniel 1:17, 20 . . . **As for these four children, God gave them knowledge and skill in all learning and wisdom . . . And in all matters of wisdom and understanding, that the king enquired of them, he found them ten times better than all the magicians and astrologers that were in all his realm.**

- 1 Corinthians 2:16 . . . **For who hath known the mind of the Lord, that he may instruct him? but we have the mind of Christ.**

- (cf. Luke 2:52; 1 Corinthians 1:30)

See also: Memory/Mental Health/Nervousness

Legs

- Deuteronomy 28:35 . . . **[Thou shalt be smitten] in the knees, and in the legs, with a sore botch that cannot be healed, from the sole of thy foot unto the top of thy head.** According to Galatians 3:13, Christ has redeemed us from leg problems.

- 1 Samuel 2:4 . . . **The bows of the mighty men are broken, and they that stumbled are girded with strength.**

- Song of Solomon 5:15 . . . **His legs are as pillars of marble, set upon sockets of fine gold: his countenance is as Lebanon, excellent as the cedars.**

- Song of Solomon 7:1 . . . **How beautiful are thy feet with shoes, O prince's daughter! the joints of thy thighs are like jewels, the work of the hands of a cunning workman.**
- Isaiah 35:6 . . . **Then shall the lame man leap as an hart, and the tongue of the dumb sing: for in the wilderness shall waters break out, and streams in the desert.**
- Zechariah 10:12 . . . **And I will strengthen them in the LORD; and they shall walk up and down in his name, saith the LORD.**
- Hebrews 12:13 . . . **And make straight paths for your feet, lest that which is lame be turned out of the way; but let it rather be healed.**

See also: Arthritis/Hips/Knees/Paralysis

Leukemia
See: Blood/Bone/ Cancer/ Hereditary Diseases/Immune System

Liver
See: Abdomen/Blood/Immune System/Jaundice/Poisoning

Lou Gehrig's Disease
See: Nervous System/Paralysis

Lungs

See: Respiratory System

Lupus

- Deuteronomy 28:61 . . . **Also every sickness, and every plague, which is not written in the book of this law . . . will [be brought] upon thee, until thou be destroyed.** According to Galatians 3:13, Christ has redeemed us from lupus.

See also: Immune System/Nervous System

Maiming Injuries

- Matthew 15:30-31 . . . **And great multitudes came unto him, having with them those that were lame, blind, dumb, maimed, and many others, and cast them down at Jesus' feet; and he healed them: insomuch that the multitude wondered, when they saw the dumb to speak, the maimed to be whole, the lame to walk, and the blind to see: and they glorified the God of Israel.**
- (cf. Luke 22:50-51)

See also: Pain/Wounds

Malaria

- Deuteronomy 28:22 . . . **[Thou shalt be smitten] with a consumption, and with a fever . . .** (*fever:* H6920 *qaddachath*-inflammation, febrile disease, and burning ague, which is a malarial disease[13]) Malaria is part of the curse; according to Galatians 3:13, Christ has redeemed us from malaria.

See also: Fever/Immune System

Malnutrition

- Deuteronomy 28:22 . . . **[Thou shalt be smitten] with a consumption** . . . (*consumption:* H7829 *shachep-heth*-emaciation which means an abnormal thinness caused by lack of nutrition or disease[3]) According to Galatians 3:13, Christ has redeemed us from emaciation.

- Psalm 22:26 . . . **The meek shall eat and be satisfied: they shall praise the LORD that seek him: your heart shall live for ever.**

- Psalm 34:8 . . . **O taste and see that the LORD is good: blessed is the man that trusteth in him.**

- Psalm 37:3 . . . **Trust in the LORD, and do good; so shalt thou dwell in the land, and verily thou shalt be fed.**

- Psalm 37:19 . . . **They shall not be ashamed in the evil time: and in the days of famine they shall be satisfied.**

- Psalm 37:25 . . . **I have been young and now am old; yet have I not seen the righteous forsaken, nor his seed begging bread.**

- Psalm 92:14 . . . They shall still bring forth fruit in old age; they shall be fat and flourishing.
- Psalm 103:5 . . . Who satisfieth thy mouth with good things; so that thy youth is renewed like the eagle's.
- Isaiah 1:19 . . . If ye be willing and obedient, ye shall eat the good of the land.
- Luke 1:53 . . . He hath filled the hungry with good things . . .
- (cf. Ecclesiastes 3:13; Daniel 1:15; Ezekiel 34:14-15; 3 John 2)

See also: Diarrhea/Underweight/Weakness

Memory
- Psalm 119:16 . . . I will delight myself in thy statutes: I will not forget thy word.
- Isaiah 11:2-3 . . . And the spirit of the LORD shall rest upon him, the spirit of wisdom and understanding, the spirit of counsel and might, the spirit of knowledge and of the fear of the LORD; and shall make him of quick understanding in the fear of the LORD. . .
- Daniel 1:17 . . . As for these four children, God gave them knowledge and skill in all learning and wisdom . . .
- John 14:26 . . . But the Comforter, which is the Holy

Ghost, whom the Father will send in my name, he shall teach you all things, and bring all things to your remembrance, whatsoever I have said unto you.

- 1 Corinthians 2:16 **. . . For who hath known the mind of the Lord, that he may instruct him? But we have the mind of Christ.**

- 2 Timothy 1:7 **. . . For God hath not given us the spirit of fear; but of power, and of love, and of a sound mind.**

See also: Mental Health

Menstrual Difficulties
See: Blood/Bone/Pain/Reproductive System

Mental and Soulical Health
- Deuteronomy 28:65 **. . . And among these nations shalt thou find no ease, neither shall the sole of thy foot have rest: but [thou shalt have] there a trembling heart, and failing of eyes, and sorrow of mind.** (*New International Version* translates *trembling heart; sorrow of mind* as *an anxious mind; a despairing heart*[6], and the *Common English Bible* renders it *agitated mind; depressed spirit*[7].) According to Galatians 3:13, Christ has redeemed us from these things.

- Psalm 23:3 **. . . He restoreth my soul: he leadeth me in the paths of righteousness for his name's sake.**

- Psalm 35:9 . . . **And my soul shall be joyful in the LORD: it shall rejoice in his salvation.**

- Psalm 138:3 . . . **In the day when I cried thou answeredst me, and strengthenedst me with strength in my soul.**

- Proverbs 4:23 . . . **Keep thy heart with all diligence; for out of it are the issues of life.**

- Romans 8:6 . . . **For to be carnally minded is death; but to be spiritually minded is life and peace.**

- Romans 12:2 . . . **And be not conformed to this world: but be ye transformed by the renewing of your mind, that ye may prove what is that good, and acceptable, and perfect will of God.**

- 1 Corinthians 2:16 . . . **For who hath known the mind of the Lord, that he may instruct him? but we have the mind of Christ.**

- Ephesians 4:22-24 . . . **That ye put off concerning the former conversation the old man, which is corrupt according to the deceitful lusts; and be renewed in the spirit of your mind; and that ye put on the new man, which after God is created in righteousness and true holiness.**

- Philippians 4:8 . . . **Finally, brethren, whatsoever things are true, whatsoever things are honest, whatsoever things are just, whatsoever things are pure,** whatsoever things are lovely, whatsoever things are of good report; if there be any virtue, and if there be any praise, think on these things.

- 1 Thessalonians 5:23 . . . And the very God of peace sanctify you wholly; and I pray God your whole spirit and soul and body be preserved blameless unto the coming of our Lord Jesus Christ.

- 2 Timothy 1:7 . . . For God hath not given us the spirit of fear; but of power, and of love, and of a sound mind.

- Hebrews 12:3 . . . For consider him that endured such contradiction of sinners against himself, lest ye be wearied and faint in your minds.

- James 1:21 . . . Wherefore lay apart all filthiness and superfluity of naughtiness, and receive with meekness the engrafted word, which is able to save your souls.

- 3 John 2 . . . Beloved, I wish above all things that thou mayest prosper and be in health, even as thy soul prospereth.

- (cf. Hebrews 4:12-13)

See also: Depression/ Learning Disability/Memory

Mouth

- Deuteronomy 28:27 . . . "[Thou shalt be smitten] with the botch of Egypt . . . (*botch:* H7822 *shechiyn* - inflammation; ulcer[1]) According to Galatians 3:13, Christ has redeemed us from the ulcers, sores and types of mouth disease.

- Psalm 51:15 . . . **O Lord, open thou my lips; and my mouth shall shew forth thy praise.**

- Psalm 81:10 . . . **I am the LORD thy God, which brought thee out of the land of Egypt: open thy mouth wide, and I will fill it.**

- Psalm 103:5 . . . **Who satisfieth thy mouth with good things; so that thy youth is renewed like the eagle's.** (Good things to speak and good things to eat!)

- Proverbs 12:18-19 . . . **The tongue of the wise is health. The lip of truth shall be established for ever . . .**

- (cf. Job 6:6; Proverbs 8:6-8; Psalm 34:8; Song of Solomon 4:3, 11; 7:9)

See also: Digestion/Jaw/Speech Disorders/Teeth

Multiple Sclerosis
See: Nervous System/Paralysis

Muscles
- Job 33:25 . . . **Let his flesh be restored *and* become fresher than in youth; let him return to the days of his youthful strength.** (AMP)

- Psalm 18:2 . . . The LORD is my rock, and my fortress, and my deliverer; my God, my strength, in whom I will trust; my buckler, and the horn of my salvation, and my high tower.
- Psalm 27:1 . . . The LORD is my light and my salvation; whom shall I fear? the LORD is the strength of my life; of whom shall I be afraid?
- (cf. Romans 8:11; 1 John 4:4)

See: Paralysis/Skin/ Specific part of the body

Neck

- Isaiah 10:27 . . . And it shall come to pass in that day, that his burden shall be taken away from off thy shoulder, and his yoke from off thy neck, and the yoke shall be destroyed because of the anointing.
- (cf. Psalm 3:3; Proverbs 29:1; Song of Solomon 4:4; 7:4; Isaiah 52:2)

See also: Back/Bones/Shoulder

Necrotizing Fasciitis (Flesh Eating Disease)

- Psalm 27:1-2 . . . The LORD is my light and my salvation; whom shall I fear? the LORD is the strength of my life; of whom shall I be afraid? When the wicked, even mine enemies and my foes, came upon me to eat up my flesh, they stumbled and fell.
- Proverbs 3:1, 8 . . . My son, do not forget my law,

but let your heart keep my commands . . . it will
be health to your flesh, and strength to your bones.
(NKJV)

- (cf. Romans 8:11; 1 John 4:4)

See also: Flesh

Nervousness

- Isaiah 26:3 . . . **Thou wilt keep him in perfect peace,
  whose mind is stayed on thee: because he trusteth in
  thee.**

- John 14:27 . . . **Peace I leave with you, my peace I
  give unto you: not as the world giveth, give I unto
  you. Let not your heart be troubled, neither let it be
  afraid.**

- Philippians 4:6 . . . **Do not fret or have any anxiety
  about anything, but in every circumstance and in
  everything, by prayer and petition (definite requests),
  with thanksgiving, continue to make your wants
  known to God.** (AMP)

- Philippians 4:7 . . . **And the peace of God, which
  passeth all understanding, shall keep your hearts and
  minds through Christ Jesus.**

- Colossians 3:15 . . . **And let the peace of God rule in
  your hearts, to the which also ye are also called in one
  body; and be ye thankful.**

- 1 Peter 5:7 . . . **Casting all your care upon him; for he careth for you.**
See also: Mental Health/Oppression/Weakness

Nervous System

- Deuteronomy 28:61 . . . **Also every sickness, and every plague, which is not written in the book of this law . . . will [be brought] upon thee, until thou be destroyed.** According to Galatians 3:13, Christ has redeemed us from any ailment of the nervous system.
- Psalm 119:165 . . . **Great peace have they which love thy law: and nothing shall offend them.**
- Proverbs 12:28 . . . **In the way of righteousness is life: and in the pathway thereof there is no death.**
- Isaiah 58:8, 12 . . . **Then shall thy light break forth as the morning, and thine health shall spring forth speedily . . . And they that shall be of thee shall build the old waste places: thou shalt raise up the foundations of many generations; and thou shalt be called, The repairer of the breach, The restorer of paths to dwell in.**
- John 1:5 . . . **The light shines in the darkness, and the darkness can never extinguish it.** (NLT)
- Philippians 4:6-7 . . . **Be careful for nothing; but in every thing by prayer and supplication with thanksgiving let your requests be made known unto God.**

And the peace of God, which passeth all understanding, shall keep your hearts and minds through Christ Jesus.

- (cf. Psalm 97:4, 11; 119:130; Proverbs 4:18; Jeremiah 32:27; Mark 9:23; Luke 1:37; 18:27. Men may say that it is impossible for nerve/brain cells to be regenerated. But the things that are impossible with men are possible with God. All things are possible to him that believes!)

See also: Memory/Mental Health

Neuritis/Neuropathy
See: Nervous System/Inflammation

Nose
- Genesis 2:7 . . . **And the LORD God formed man of the dust of the ground, and breathed into his nostrils the breath of life; and man became a living soul.**
- (cf. Song of Solomon 7:4, 8)

See also: Respiratory System

Numbness
See: Nervous System/Paralysis

Obesity/Overweight
- Proverbs 18:20 . . . **A man's belly shall be satisfied with the fruit of his mouth; and with the increase of his**

lips shall he be filled.

- Proverbs 23: 20-21 . . . Be not among winebibbers; among riotous eaters of flesh: for the drunkard and the glutton shall come to poverty: and drowsiness shall clothe a man with rags.

- 1 Corinthians 6:12 . . . All things are lawful unto me, but all things are not expedient: all things are lawful for me, but I will not be brought under the power of any.

- 1 Corinthians 9:27 . . . But I keep under my body, and bring it into subjection: lest that by any means, when I have preached to others, I myself should be a castaway.

- Galatians 5:16 . . . This I say then, Walk in the Spirit, and ye shall not fulfil the lust of the flesh.

- (cf. Proverbs 23:1-3; Matthew 17:21)

Oppression

- Nehemiah 8:10 . . . Then he said unto them, Go your way, eat the fat, and drink the sweet, and send portions unto them for whom nothing is prepared: for this day is holy unto our LORD: neither be ye sorry; for the joy of the LORD is your strength.

- Psalm 72:4 . . . He shall judge the poor of the people, he shall save the children of the needy, and shall break in pieces the oppressor.

- Psalm 103:6 . . . The LORD executeth righteousness and judgment for all that are oppressed.

- Isaiah 9:4 . . . For thou has broken the yoke of his burden, and the staff of his shoulder, the rod of his oppressor, as in the day of Midian.

- Isaiah 10:27 . . . And it shall come to pass in that day, that his burden shall be taken away from off thy shoulder, and his yoke from off thy neck, and the yoke shall be destroyed because of the anointing.

- Isaiah 14:2 . . . And the people shall take them, and bring them to their place: and the house of Israel shall possess them in the land of the LORD for servants and handmaids: and they shall take them captives, whose captives they were; and they shall rule over their oppressors.

- Isaiah 52:2 . . . Shake thyself from the dust; arise, and sit down, O Jerusalem: loose thyself from the bands of thy neck, O captive daughter of Zion.

- Isaiah 54:14-15 . . . In righteousness shalt thou be established: thou shalt be far from oppression; for thou shalt not fear: and from terror; for it shall not come near thee. Behold, they shall surely gather together, but not by me: whosoever shall gather together against thee shall fall for thy sake.

- Zechariah 9:8 . . . **And I will encamp about mine house because of the army, because of him that passeth by, and because of him that returneth: and no oppressor shall pass through them any more: for now have I seen with mine eyes.**

- Philippians 4:6 . . . **Do not fret or have any anxiety about anything, but in every circumstance and in everything, by prayer and petition (definite requests), with thanksgiving, continue to make your wants known to God.** (AMP)

- James 4:7 . . . **Submit yourselves therefore to God. Resist the devil, and he will flee from you.**

- (cf. Matthew 4:24; Luke 10:19; 13:11-16)

See also: Depression

Osteoporosis

- Job 21:24 . . . **His pails are full of milk, and the marrow of his bones is moist.** (NKJV)

- Psalm 118:14 . . . **The LORD is my strength and song, and is become my salvation.**

- Proverbs 3:8 . . . **It [God's law] will be health to your flesh, and strength to your bones.** (NKJV)

- Isaiah 58:11 . . . **The LORD will guide you continually, and satisfy your soul in drought, and strengthen your bones; you shall be like a watered garden,** and like a spring of water, whose waters do not fail. (NKJV)

- Ezekiel 37:3-5 . . . **And He said to me, "Son of man, can these bones live?" So I answered, "O Lord GOD, You know." Again He said to me, "Prophesy to these bones, and say to them, 'O dry bones, hear the word of the LORD! Thus says the Lord GOD to these bones: "Surely I will cause breath to enter into you, and you shall live."'"** (NKJV)

- (cf. 2 Kings 13:21; Job 10:11-12; Proverbs 12:4; 14:30; 15:30; 17:22; Jeremiah 20:9)

See also: Bones

Ovary

See: Abdomen/Barrenness/Reproductive System

Pain

- Isaiah 53:4 . . . **Surely He has borne our griefs (sicknesses, weaknesses, and distresses) and carried our sorrows and pains [of punishment]** . . . (AMP)

- Matthew 4:24 . . . **News about him spread all over Syria, and people brought to him all who were ill with various diseases, those suffering severe pain, the demon-possessed, those having seizures, and the paralyzed; and he healed them.** (NIV)

Palsy

- Matthew 4:24 . . . **And his fame went throughout all Syria: and they brought unto him all sick people that were taken with divers diseases and torments, and those which were possessed with devils, and those which were lunatick, and those that had the palsy; and he healed them.**

- Matthew 8:5-7, 13 . . . **And when Jesus was entered into Capernaum, there came unto him a centurion, beseeching him, and saying, Lord, my servant lieth at home sick of the palsy, grievously tormented. And Jesus saith unto him, I will come and heal him... And Jesus said unto the centurion, Go thy way; and as thou hast believed, so be it done unto thee. And his servant was healed in the selfsame hour.**

- Acts 9:33-34 . . . **And there he found a certain man named Aeneas, which had kept his bed eight years, and was sick of the palsy. And Peter said unto him, Aeneas, Jesus Christ maketh thee whole: arise, and make thy bed. And he arose immediately.**

See also: Paralysis

Panic Attack

- Deuteronomy 28:65 . . . **And among these nations shalt thou find no ease, neither shall the sole of thy foot have rest: but [thou shalt have] there a trembling** heart, and failing of eyes, and sorrow of mind. (*New International Version* translates *trembling heart; sorrow of mind* as *an anxious mind; a despairing heart*[6], and the *Common English Bible* renders it *agitated mind; depressed spirit*[7].) According to Galatians 3:13, Christ has redeemed us from these panic attacks.

- Psalm 34:19 . . . **Many are the afflictions of the righteous: but the LORD delivereth him out of them all.**

- Proverbs 3:25 . . . **Have no fear of sudden disaster or of the ruin that overtakes the wicked, for the LORD will be at your side and will keep your foot from being snared. (NIV)**

- Isaiah 51:13 . . . **Yet you have forgotten the LORD, your Creator, the one who stretched out the sky like a canopy and laid the foundations of the earth. Will you remain in constant dread of human oppressors? Will you continue to fear the anger of your enemies? Where is their fury and anger now? It is gone! (NLT)**

- Romans 8:6 . . . **For to be carnally minded is death; but to be spiritually minded is life and peace.**

See also: Fear/Nervousness/Oppression

Paralysis

- Isaiah 35:6 . . . **Then shall the lame man leap as an hart, and the tongue of the dumb sing: for in the wilderness shall waters break out, and streams in the desert.**

- Matthew 4:24 . . . So his fame spread throughout all Syria, and they brought him all the sick, those afflicted with various diseases and pains, those oppressed by demons, epileptics, and paralytics, and he healed them. (ESV)

- Matthew 8:5-8, 13 . . . When Jesus returned to Capernaum, a Roman officer came and pleaded with him, "Lord, my young servant lies in bed, paralyzed and in terrible pain." Jesus said, "I will come and heal him." But the officer said, "Lord, I am not worthy to have you come into my home. Just say the word from where you are, and my servant will be healed. Then Jesus said to the Roman officer, "Go back home. Because you believed, it has happened." And the young servant was healed that same hour. (NLT)

- Matthew 15:30 . . . And great multitudes came unto him, having with them those that were lame, blind, dumb, maimed, and many others, and cast them down at Jesus' feet; and he healed them.

- Luke 7:22 . . . Then Jesus answering said unto them, Go your way, and tell John what things ye have seen and heard; how that the blind see, the lame walk, the lepers are cleansed, the deaf hear, the dead are raised, to the poor the gospel is preached.

- (cf. Matthew 4:24; Matthew 9:2-7; Mark 2:2-12; Luke 5:18-25; John 5:5-9; Acts 3:2-8; 9:33-34; 14:8-10)

See also: Hips/Knees/Legs/Nervous System/Palsy

Parasites

- Exodus 11:7 . . . **But against any of the children of Israel shall not a dog move his tongue, against man or beast: that ye may know how that the LORD doth put a difference between the Egyptians and Israel.**

- Deuteronomy 28:21 . . . **Pestilence [shall] cleave unto thee, until [it has] consumed thee from off the land, whither thou goest to possess it.** According to Galatians 3:13, Christ has redeemed us from pestilence.

- Psalm 3:3 . . . **But thou, O LORD, art a shield for me; my glory, and the lifter up of mine head.**

- Psalm 91:3, 10 . . . **Surely he shall deliver thee from the snare of the fowler, and from the noisome pestilence. There shall no evil befall thee, neither shall any plague come nigh thy dwelling.**

- Proverbs 30:5 . . . **Every word of God is pure: he is a shield unto them that put their trust in him.**

- Isaiah 4:5 . . . **And the LORD will create upon every dwelling place of mount Zion, and upon her assemblies, a cloud and smoke by day, and the shining of flaming fire by night: for upon all the glory shall be a defence.**

- Romans 8:2 . . . **For the law of the Spirit of life in Christ Jesus hath made me free from the law of sin**

and death.

- (cf. Luke 10:19)

Parkinson's Disease

See: Nervous System/Palsy/Paralysis

Phobia

See: Fear/Nervousness/Oppression/Panic Attack

Pneumonia

See: Immune System/Respiratory System

Poisoning

- Exodus 23:25 . . . **And ye shall serve the LORD your God, and he shall bless thy bread, and thy water; and I will take sickness away from the midst of thee.**
- Mark 16:18 . . . **They shall take up serpents; and if they drink any deadly thing, it shall not hurt them; they shall lay hands on the sick, and they shall recover.**
- Luke 10:19 . . . **Behold, I give unto you power to tread on serpents and scorpions, and over all the power of the enemy: and nothing shall by any means hurt you.**
- (cf. 2 Kings 4:38-41; Psalm 91:3, 6-10)

See also: Abdomen/Diarrhea/Snakebite

Polio

See: Immune System/Nervous System/Paralysis

Prostate

See: Groin/Legs

Rabies

See: Zoonosis

Rash

See: Itch

Reproductive System

- Genesis 49:25 . . . **Even by the God of thy father, who shall help thee; and by the Almighty, who shall bless thee with blessings of heaven above, blessings of the deep that lieth under, blessings of the breasts, and of the womb.**

- Exodus 23:26 . . . **There shall nothing cast their young, nor be barren, in thy land: the number of thy days I will fulfil.**

- Deuteronomy 28:18 . . . **Cursed shall be the fruit of thy body.** According to Galatians 3:13, Christ has redeemed us from the curse of miscarriages.

- Proverbs 3:8 . . . **It [God's law] shall be health to thy navel, and marrow to thy bones.** (*navel*: H8270 *shor-*

umbilical cord[14])

- Proverbs 18:20 . . . A man's belly shall be satisfied with the fruit of his mouth; and with the increase of his lips shall he be filled. (*belly:* H990 *beten-* the belly, especially the womb[15])

- Malachi 3:11 . . . And I will rebuke the devourer for your sakes, and he shall not destroy the fruits of your ground; neither shall your vine cast her fruit before the time in the field, saith the LORD of hosts.

- Galatians 3:9, 13-14 . . . So then they which be of faith are blessed with faithful Abraham. Christ hath redeemed us from the curse of the law, being made a curse for us: for it is written, Cursed is every one that hangeth on a tree: that the blessing of Abraham might come on the Gentiles through Jesus Christ; that we might receive the promise of the Spirit through faith.

- (cf. Luke 8:43-48)

See also: Barrenness/Hereditary Diseases

Respiratory System
- Genesis 2:7 . . . And the LORD God formed man of the dust of the ground, and breathed into his nostrils the breath of life; and man became a living soul.

- Isaiah 42:5 . . . Thus saith God the LORD, he that created the heavens, and stretched them out; he that spread forth the earth, and that which cometh out of it; he that giveth breath unto the people upon it, and spirit to them that walk therein.

- Ezekiel 37:5 . . . Thus saith the Lord GOD unto these bones: Behold, I will cause breath to enter into you, and ye shall live.

- Acts 17:25 . . . Neither is [God] worshipped with men's hands, as though he needed any thing, seeing he giveth to all life, breath, and all things.

Resuscitation

- Psalm 118:17 . . . I shall not die, but live, and declare the works of the LORD.

- Ezekiel 37:5 . . . Thus saith the Lord GOD unto these bones; Behold, I will cause breath to enter into you, and ye shall live.

- Matthew 10:7-8 . . . And as ye go, preach, saying, The kingdom of heaven is at hand. Heal the sick, cleanse the lepers, raise the dead, cast out devils: freely ye have received, freely give.

- 1 Corinthians 15:55 . . . O death, where is thy sting? O grave, where is thy victory?

- Hebrews 2:14-15 . . . Forasmuch then as the children are partakers of flesh and blood, he also himself likewise took part of the same; that through death he might destroy him that had the power of death, that is, the devil. And deliver them who through fear of death were all their lifetime subject to bondage.

- (cf. 1 Kings 17:17-23; 2 Kings 4:32-37; 13:20-21; Matthew 9:23-25; Mark 5:23, 35-43; Luke 7:11-15; John 11:38-44; Acts 9:38-41; 14:19-20; 20:9-12)

Rosacea

See: Skin/Rash

Scabies

See: Itch

Scurvy (Vitamin C Deficiency)

- Deuteronomy 28:27 . . . [Thou shalt be smitten] with the botch of Egypt, and with the emerods, and with the scab... (*scab:* H1618 *garab*-scurvy[16]) According to Galatians 3:13, Christ has redeemed us from scurvy and all vitamin deficiencies.

See also: Malnutrition

Seizures

- Matthew 4:24 . . . News about him spread all over Syria, and people brought to him all who were ill with various diseases, those suffering severe pain, the demon-possessed, those having seizures, and the

paralyzed; and he healed them. (NIV)

See: Epilepsy/Mental Health/Nervous System/Oppression

Shoulder

- Psalm 81:6 . . . **I removed his shoulder from the burden: his hands were delivered from the pots.**

- Isaiah 9:4 . . . **For thou hast broken the yoke of his burden, and the staff of his shoulder, the rod of his oppressor, as in the day of Midian.**

- Isaiah 10:27 . . . **His burden shall be taken away from off thy shoulder, and his yoke from off thy neck, and the yoke shall be destroyed because of the anointing.**

- (cf. Deuteronomy 33:12;Isaiah 14:24-26)

See also: Bones/Skin

Sinus Conditions

See: Immune System/Respiratory System

Skin

- Deuteronomy 28:27 . . . **[Thou shalt be smitten] with the botch of Egypt, and with the emerods, and with the scab, and with the itch, whereof thou canst be healed.** (*botch:* H7822 *shechiyn*-boil, inflammation[1]; *emerods:* H2914 *techor*-tumors[9]; *scab:* H1618 *garab*-itch, scab[16]; *itch:* H2275 *cherec*-skin eruptions[17]) According to Galatians 3:13, Christ has redeemed us from all manner of skin disease.

- Job 33:25 . . . His flesh shall be restored *and* become fresher than in youth. (AMP)
- Job 10:11-12 . . . Thou hast clothed me with skin and flesh, and hast fenced me with bones and sinews. Thou hast granted me life and favour, and thy visitation hath preserved my spirit.

See also: Acne/Eczema/Rash/Wounds

Sleep Disorders
- 1 Kings 8:56 . . . Blessed be the LORD, that hath given rest unto his people Israel, according to all that he promised: there hath not failed one word of all his good promise, which he promised by the hand of Moses his servant.
- Psalm 3:5 . . . I laid me down and slept; I awakened; for the LORD sustained me.
- Psalm 4:8 . . . I will both lay me down in peace, and sleep: for thou, O LORD, only makest me dwell in safety.
- Psalm 23:2 . . . He maketh me to lie down in green pastures: he leadeth me beside the still waters.
- Psalm 16:7 . . . I will praise the Lord, who counsels me; even at night my heart instructs me.
- Psalm 127:2 . . . The Lord provides for those he loves, even while they are sleeping. (ERV) (Ephesians 1:6 says that we are well accepted in the beloved!)

- Proverbs 3:24 . . . When thou liest down, thou shalt not be afraid: yea, thou shalt lie down, and thy sleep shall be sweet.

- Isaiah 32:18 . . . And my people shall dwell in a peaceable habitation, and in sure dwellings, and in quiet resting places.

Snakebite

- Genesis 1:26-28 . . . And God said, Let us make man in our image, after our likeness: and let them have dominion over the fish of the sea, and over the fowl of the air, and over the cattle, and over all the earth, and over every creeping thing that creepeth upon the earth. So God created man in his own image, in the image of God created he him; male and female created he them. And God blessed them, and God said unto them, Be fruitful, and multiply, and replenish the earth, and subdue it: and have dominion over the fish of the sea, and over the fowl of the air, and over every living thing that moveth upon the earth.

- Psalm 91:13 . . . Thou shalt tread upon the lion and adder: the young lion and the dragon shall thou trample under feet.

- Mark 16:18 . . . They shall take up serpents; and if they drink any deadly thing, it shall not hurt them; they shall lay hands on the sick, and they shall recover.

- Luke 10:19 . . . Behold, I give unto you power to tread

on serpents and scorpions, and over all the power of the enemy: and nothing shall by any means hurt you.

- Philippians 2:9-10 . . . Wherefore God also hath highly exalted him, and given him a name which is above every name: that at the name of Jesus every knee should bow, of things in heaven, and things in earth, and things under the earth.
- (cf. Genesis 3:14-15; Exodus 4:2-4; 7:10-12; Numbers 21:8-9; Acts 28:3-6)

See also: Poisoning

Speech Impediments and Disorders
- Psalm 45:1 . . . My tongue is the pen of a ready writer.
- Isaiah 32:4 . . . The heart also of the rash shall understand knowledge, and the tongue of the stammerers shall be ready to speak plainly.
- Isaiah 35:6 . . . Then shall the lame man leap as an hart, and the tongue of the dumb sing: for in the wilderness shall waters break out, and streams in the desert.
- Isaiah 50:4... The Lord GOD hath given me the tongue of the learned, that I should know how to speak a word in season to him that is weary: he wakeneth morning by morning, he wakeneth mine ear to hear as the learned.
- Mark 7:32-35 . . . And they bring unto him one that

was deaf, and had an impediment in his speech; and
they beseech him to put his hand upon him. And
he took him aside from the multitude, and put his
fingers into his ears, and he spit, and touched his
tongue; and looking up to heaven, he sighed, and
saith unto him, Ephphatha, that is, Be opened. And
straightway his ears were opened, and the string of
his tongue was loosed, and he spake plain.

- (cf. Exodus 4:10-12; Song of Solomon 4:3; Jeremiah
  1:6-9; Matthew 9:32-33; 12:34-37; Colossians 4:3-6)

Stomach

- Mark 16:18 . . . They shall take up serpents; and if
  they drink any deadly thing, it shall not hurt them;
  they shall lay hands on the sick, and they shall recover.

- Luke 10:19 . . . Behold, I give unto you power to tread
  on serpents and scorpions, and over all the power of
  the enemy: and nothing shall by any means hurt you.

- (cf. Psalm 34:8,10; 103:5; Matthew 6:26; 15:17; 1 Corinthians 4:8)

See also: Abdomen

Stress

- Matthew 6:25-34 . . . Therefore I say unto you, Take
  no thought for your life, what ye shall eat, or what ye
  shall drink; nor yet for your body, what ye shall put
  on. Is not the life more than meat, and the body than

raiment? Behold the fowls of the air: for they sow not, neither do they reap, nor gather into barns; yet your heavenly Father feedeth them. Are ye not much better than they? Which of you by taking thought can add one cubit unto his stature? And why take ye thought for raiment? Consider the lilies of the field, how they grow; they toil not, neither do they spin: and yet I say unto you, That even Solomon in all his glory was not arrayed like one of these. Wherefore, if God so clothe the grass of the field, which to day is, and to morrow is cast into the oven, shall he not much more clothe you, O ye of little faith? Therefore take no thought, saying, What shall we eat? or, What shall we drink? or, Wherewithal shall we be clothed? (For after all these things do the Gentiles seek:) for your heavenly Father knoweth that ye have need of all these things. But seek ye first the kingdom of God, and his righteousness; and all these things shall be added unto you. Take therefore no thought for the morrow: for the morrow shall take thought for the things of itself. Sufficient unto the day is the evil thereof.

- 1 Peter 5:7 . . . **Casting all your care upon him; for he careth for you.**

See: Mental Health/Nervousness/Oppression/Worry

Stroke

- Deuteronomy 28:59 . . . **Then hath Jehovah made wonderful thy strokes, and the strokes of thy seed - great strokes, and stedfast, and evil sickness, and stedfast.** (YLT) Strokes are part of the curse; according to Galatians 3:13, Christ has redeemed us from strokes.

See also: Blood/Nervous System/Sunstroke

Sunburn

- Deuteronomy 28:27 . . . **[Thou shalt be smitten] with the botch of Egypt, and with the emerods, and with the scab, and with the itch, whereof thou canst be healed.** (*itch:* H2275 *cherec*-skin eruptions[17]) According to Galatians 3:13, Christ has redeemed us from sunburn.

- Psalm 121:5-6 . . . **The LORD is thy keeper: the LORD is thy shade upon thy right hand. The sun shall not smite thee by day, nor the moon by night.**

- Isaiah 49:10 . . . **They shall not hunger nor thirst; neither shall the heat nor sun smite them: for he that hath mercy on them shall lead them, even by the springs of water shall he guide them.**

- (cf. Genesis 15:1)

Sunstroke

- Deuteronomy 28:22 . . . **[Thou shalt be smitten] with a consumption, and with a fever, and with an inflammation, and with an extreme burning** . . . (*extreme* *burning:* H2746 *charchur*-extreme heat, inflammation, violent heat, fever[18]) According to Galatians 3:13, Christ has redeemed us from sunstroke.

See also: Stroke

Systematic Lupus Erythematosus

- Deuteronomy 28:61 . . . **Also every sickness, and every plague, which is not written in the book of this law . . . will [be brought] upon thee, until thou be destroyed.** According to Galatians 3:13, Christ has redeemed us from Systematic Lupus Erythematosus.

See also: Immune System/Specific part of the body

Tastebuds

See: Mouth

Teeth

- Song of Solomon 4:2 . . . **Thy teeth are like a flock of sheep that are even shorn, which came up from the washing; whereof every one bear twins, and none is barren among them.**

See also: Bones/Mouth

Tetanus

See: Immune System/Jaw

Tongue

- Proverbs 12:18 . . . **There is that speaketh like the piercings of a sword: but the tongue of the wise is health.**

- (cf. Song of Solomon 4:11)

See also: Mouth

Tonsillitis

- Deuteronomy 28:61 . . . **Also every sickness, and every plague, which is not written in the book of this law . . . will [be brought] upon thee, until thou be destroyed.** According to Galatians 3:13, Christ has redeemed us from tonsillitis.

See also: Immune System

Tuberculosis

- Deuteronomy 28:22 . . . **[Thou shalt be smitten] with a consumption . . .** (*consumption:* H7829 *shachepheth*-emaciation; wasting disease of the lungs[3]) According to Galatians 3:13, Christ has redeemed us from tuberculosis.

See also: Immune System/Respiratory System/Skin

Tumors

- Deuteronomy 28:27 . . . **[You will be smitten] with the botch of Egypt, and with the emerods . . .** (*emerods:*

H2914 *techor*-tumors, hemorrhoids, piles[9]) According to Galatians 3:13, Christ has redeemed us from tumors.

- Deuteronomy 28:59 . . . **Then the LORD will bring on you and your offspring extraordinary afflictions, afflictions severe and lasting, and sicknesses grievous and lasting.** (ESV) Tumors and cancer are part of the curse; according to Galatians 3:13, Christ has redeemed us from tumors, growths, abnormal lumps, cysts, and warts.

See also: Cancer/Skin/Specific part of the body

Typhoid
See: Immune System/Fever

Ulcers
- Deuteronomy 28:27 . . . **[You will be smitten] with the botch of Egypt . . .** (*botch:* H7822 *shechiyn*-inflammation, boil or ulcer[1]) According to Galatians 3:13, Christ has redeemed us from ulcers.

See also: Mouth/Skin

Urinary Tract
See: Kidneys

Veins
- Deuteronomy 28:61 . . . **Also every sickness, and every plague, which is not written in the book of this law...**

will [be brought] upon thee, until thou be destroyed.
According to Galatians 3:13, Christ has redeemed us
from any ailment of the veins.

See also: Blood

Virus
See: Blood/Immune System

Warts

- Matthew 15:13 . . . **But he answered and said, Every
plant, which my heavenly Father hath not planted,
shall be rooted up.**

See also: Tumors

Weakness

- Job 23:6 . . . **Will he plead against me with his great
power? No; but he would put strength in me.**

- Psalm 27:1 . . . **The LORD is my light and salvation;
whom shall I fear? the LORD is the strength of my
life; of whom shall I be afraid?**

- Psalm 68:28, 35 . . . **Thy God hath commanded thy
strength: strengthen, O God, that which thou hast
wrought for us . . . the God of Israel is he that giveth
strength and power unto his people. Blessed be God.**

- Joel 3:10 . . . **Beat your plowshares into swords and**

your pruninghooks into spears: let the weak say, I am strong.

- Romans 8:11 . . . But if the Spirit of him that raised up Jesus from the dead dwell in you, he that raised up Christ from the dead shall also quicken your mortal bodies by his Spirit that dwelleth in you.

- Romans 8:26 . . . In the same way, the Spirit helps us in our weakness... (NIV)

- 2 Corinthians 12:9-10 . . . And he said unto me, My grace is sufficient for thee: for my strength is made perfect in weakness.

- Ephesians 3:16 . . . That he would grant you, according to the riches of his glory, to be strengthened with might by his Spirit in the inner man.

- Ephesians: 6:10 . . . Finally, my brethren, be strong in the Lord, and in the power of his might.

- Philippians 4:13 . . . I can do all things through Christ which strengtheneth me.

- (cf. Psalm 18:29, 32; 28:7; 29:11; 71:16; 73:26; 84:4-7; 105:4; 138:3; Isaiah 26:4; 40:28-31; 41:10; Zechariah 10:12)

Worry

- Isaiah 26:3 . . . Thou wilt keep him in perfect peace, whose mind is stayed on thee: because he trusteth in thee.

- Isaiah 32:18 . . . **And my people shall dwell in a peaceful habitation, and in sure dwellings, and in quiet resting places.**

- Matthew 6:25-34 . . . Therefore I tell you, do not worry about your life, what you will eat or drink; or about your body, what you will wear. Is not life more than food, and the body more than clothes? Look at the birds of the air; they do not sow or reap or store away in barns, and yet your heavenly Father feeds them. Are you not much more valuable than they? Can any one of you by worrying add a single hour to your life? And why do you worry about clothes? See how the flowers of the field grow. They do not labor or spin. Yet I tell you that not even Solomon in all his splendor was dressed like one of these. If that is how God clothes the grass of the field, which is here today and tomorrow is thrown into the fire, will he not much more clothe you - you of little faith? So do not worry, saying, 'What shall we eat?' or 'What shall we drink?' or 'What shall we wear?' For the pagans run after all these things, and your heavenly Father knows that you need them. But seek first his kingdom and his righteousness, and all these things will be given to you as well. Therefore do not worry about tomorrow, for tomorrow will worry about itself. Each day has enough trouble of its own. (NIV)

- Philippians 4:6-7 . . . **Do not be anxious about any-thing, but in every situation, by prayer and petition, with thanksgiving, present your requests to God. And the peace of God, which transcends all understand-ing, will guard your hearts and your minds in Christ Jesus.** (NIV)
- 1 Peter 5:7 . . . **Casting all your care upon him; for he careth for you.**

Wounds

- Psalm 147:3 . . . **He healeth the broken in heart, and bindeth up their wounds.**
- Isaiah 53:5 . . . **But he was wounded for our transgres-sions, he was bruised for our iniquities: the chastise-ment of our peace was upon him; and with his stripes we are healed.**
- Jeremiah 30:17 . . . **For I will restore health unto thee, and I will heal thee of thy wounds, saith the LORD. . .**
- Ezekiel 34:16 . . . **[I] will bind up that which was bro-ken, and will strengthen that which was sick . . .**
- Matthew 15:30 . . . **And great multitudes came unto him, having with them those that were lame, blind, dumb, maimed, and many others, and cast them down at Jesus' feet; and he healed them.**

- Luke 22:50-51 . . . **And one of them smote the servant of the high priest, and cut off his right ear. And Jesus answered and said, Suffer ye thus far. And he touched his ear, and healed him.**

See also: Pain

Wrist
See: Arthritis/Hands

X, Y, Z (Male and Female Chromosomes, Zygote-Fertilized Egg)
See: Hereditary Diseases/Reproductive System

Xanthoma
See: Skin/Tumors

Xerophthalmia
See: Eyes

Zoonosis

- Exodus 11:7 . . . **But against any of the children of Israel shall not a dog move his tongue, against man or beast: that ye may know how that the LORD doth put a difference between the Egyptians and Israel.**
- Psalm 22:12-13, 20-21 . . . **Many bulls have compassed me: strong bulls of Bashan have beset me round. They gaped upon me with their mouths, as a**

ravening and a roaring lion. Deliver my soul from the sword; my darling from the power of the dog. Save me from the lion's mouth: for thou hast heard me . . .

- Daniel 6:22 . . . My God hath sent his angel, and hath shut the lions' mouths, that they have not hurt me . . .

- (cf. Leviticus 26:22)

See also: Immune System/Seizure/Snakebites

Appendix Four

Helpful Study Resources

"**L**ET THEM NOT DEPART FROM thine eyes; keep them in the midst of thine heart. For they are life unto those that find them, and health to all their flesh.**"** (Proverbs 4:21-22) It is so important to keep the Word of God in your ears and before your eyes, even before symptoms of sickness touch your body. Here are some absolute must-have resources for every doctor, nurse, and born again believer, tools and materials to help you keep your focus on the Healer, Jesus Christ. These great teachings will light your fire even if your wood is wet!

Books and CD Series

Christ the Healer by F.F. Bosworth

Spiritual Gifts and Their Operation by Howard Carter

God's Plan for Man by Finis Jennings Dake

Bible Truths Unmasked by Finis Jennings Dake

Gifts of the Holy Spirit by Kenneth E. Hagin

Health Food Devotions by Kenneth E. Hagin

God's Healing Word by Trina Hankins

How To Receive Divine Healing by Mark and Trina Hankins

God's Word for Your Healing by Harrison House

God's Healing Promises by Charles and Frances Hunter

Handbook for Healing by Charles and Frances Hunter

Jesus the Healer by E.W. Kenyon

Supernatural Childbirth by Jackie Mize

Healing the Sick by T.L. Osborn

Healed of Cancer by Dodie Osteen

Sparkling Gems: From the Greek by Rick Renner

Miracles: Eyewitness to the Miraculous by R. W. Schambach

You Can't Beat God Givin' by R. W. Schambach

The Anointing for Miracles by R.W. Schambach & Donna
Schambach

The Gifts and Ministries of the Holy Spirit by Lester Sumrall

Ever Increasing Faith by Smith Wigglesworth

✶✶✶✶✶

Websites

Charles Capps Ministries
http://cappsministries.com/pages/media-center
Kenneth Copeland Ministries
www.kcm.org/real-help/healing
Jesse Duplantis Ministries
http://www.jdm.org/xw-magazine.aspx
Kenneth Hagin Ministries
"Health Food Devotional" www.rhema.org/?option=com_
healthfood&Itemid=19
Keith Moore Ministries
Free downloads on healing at www.moorelife.org
Rick Renner Ministries
www.renner.org
Jerry Savelle Ministries
http://www.jerrysavelle.org/media/aif/

*****

Links

http://www.renner.org/healing/is-there-any-sick-among-you/

http://www.renner.org/healing/scourged/

http://www.renner.org/healing/they-shall-lay-hands-on-the-sick/

https://www.cfan.org.uk/gospel-campaigns/testimonies

Citations

Chapter One

1. "G4991 - sōtēria - Strong's Greek Lexicon (KJV)." Blue Letter Bible. Web. 19 Jul, 2016.

Chapter Two

1. "G2098 - euaggelion - Strong's Greek Lexicon (KJV)." Blue Letter Bible. Web. 24 Aug, 2016.

2. "G1242 - diathēkē - Strong's Greek Lexicon (KJV)." Blue Letter Bible. Web. 24 Aug, 2016.

Chapter Three

1. "H7829 - shachepheth - Strong's Hebrew Lexicon (KJV)." Blue Letter Bible. Web. 25 Aug, 2016.

2. "BibleGateway." *Deut 28:22 TLB*. N.p., n.d. Web. 25 Aug. 2016.

3. "BibleGateway." *Deut 28:22 GNT*. N.p., n.d. Web. 25 Aug. 2016.

4. "H6920 - qaddachath - Strong's Hebrew Lexicon (KJV)." Blue Letter Bible. Web. 25 Aug, 2016.

5. "H1816 - dalleqeth - Strong's Hebrew Lexicon (KJV)." Blue Letter Bible. Web. 25 Aug, 2016.

6. "BibleGateway." *Deut 28:22 NET*. N.p., n.d. Web. 25 Aug. 2016.

7. "BibleGateway." *Deut 28:22 NLV*. N.p., n.d. Web. 25 Aug. 2016.

8. "H2719 - chereb - Strong's Hebrew Lexicon (KJV)." Blue Letter Bible. Web. 25 Aug, 2016.

9. "H3420 - yeraqown - Strong's Hebrew Lexicon (KJV)." Blue Letter Bible. Web. 25 Aug, 2016.

10. "H7822 - shĕchiyn - Strong's Hebrew Lexicon (KJV)." Blue Letter Bible. Web. 25 Aug, 2016.

11. "H2914 - tĕchor - Strong's Hebrew Lexicon (KJV)." Blue Letter Bible. Web. 25 Aug, 2016.

12. "Knox Bible." *Knox Bible*. N.p., n.d. Web. 25 Aug. 2016.

13. "H1618 - garab - Strong's Hebrew Lexicon (KJV)." Blue Letter Bible. Web. 25 Aug, 2016.

14. "BibleGateway." *Deut 28:27 NET*. N.p., n.d. Web. 25 Aug. 2016.

15. "BibleGateway." *Deut 28:28 CJB*. N.p., n.d. Web. 25 Aug. 2016.

16. "BibleGateway." *Deut 28:28 GNT*. N.p., n.d. Web. 25 Aug. 2016.

17. "BibleGateway." *Deut 28:28 CEB*. N.p., n.d. Web. 25

Aug. 2016.

18. "H8541 - timmahown - Strong's Hebrew Lexicon (KJV)." Blue Letter Bible. Web. 25 Aug, 2016.

19. "BibleGateway." *Deut 28:28 NIV.* N.p., n.d. Web. 25 Aug. 2016.

20. "BibleGateway." *Deut 28:28 TLB.* N.p., n.d. Web. 25 Aug. 2016.

21. "BibleGateway." *Deut 28:59 YLT.* N.p., n.d. Web. 26 Aug. 2016.

22. "BibleGateway." *Deut 28:59 GNT.* N.p., n.d. Web. 26 Aug. 2016.

23. "BibleGateway." *Deut 28:59 NASB.* N.p., n.d. Web. 26 Aug. 2016.

24. "BibleGateway." *Deut 28:59 NABRE.* N.p., n.d. Web. 26 Aug. 2016.

25. "BibleGateway." *Deut 28:59 AMPC.* N.p., n.d. Web. 26 Aug. 2016.

26. "BibleGateway." *Deut 28:65 NIV.* N.p., n.d. Web. 26 Aug. 2016.

27. "BibleGateway." *Deut 28:65 CEB.* N.p., n.d. Web. 26 Aug. 2016.

Chapter Four

1. "H1897 - hagah - Strong's Hebrew Lexicon (KJV)." Blue Letter Bible. Web. 30 Aug, 2016.

Chapter Seven

1. Winborn, Tracy. "Reopening the Wells: Legacy of Lake's Healing Rooms." *CBN.com (beta)*. N.p., 08 Sept. 2014. Web. 13 Dec. 2016.

Chapter Nine

1. Winston, Bill, Dr. "Confession for Divine Health." *Prayers and Confessions | Living Word Christian Center*. N.p., n.d. Web. 13 Jan. 2017.

2. Moore, Keith. "A Faith Confession." *Moore Life Ministries - Branson, MO*. N.p., n.d. Web. 13 Jan. 2017.

3. Hankins, Trina. *God's Healing Word*. Alexandria: Mark Hankins Ministries, 2013. 128. Print.

Appendix One

1. "Etymology." *Merriam-Webster.com*. Merriam-Webster, n.d. Web. 12 July 2016.

2. "Student Dictionary." *Word Central*. Meriam-Webster, n.d. Web.

3. Strong, James. *Strong's Exhaustive Concordance*. Peabody, MA: Hendrickson, 1007. Print.

4. Bauer, Walter. *A Greek-English Lexicon of the New Testament*. Chicago: U of Chicago, 1952. Print.

5. Bauer, Walter. *A Greek-English Lexicon of the New Testament*. Chicago: U of Chicago, 1957. Print.

6. "H7495 - rapha' - Strong's Hebrew Lexicon (KJV)."
   Blue Letter Bible. Web. 15 Jul, 2016.

7. "H7500 - riph'uwth - Strong's Hebrew Lexicon (KJV)."
   Blue Letter Bible. Web. 15 Jul, 2016.

8. "H4832 ·· marpe' - Strong's Hebrew Lexicon (KJV)."
   Blue Letter Bible. Web. 15 Jul, 2016.

9. "H7965 - shalowm - Strong's Hebrew Lexicon (KJV)."
   Blue Letter Bible. Web. 15 Jul, 2016.

10. "H3444 - yĕshuw`ah - Strong's Hebrew Lexicon (KJV)."
    Blue Letter Bible. Web. 15 Jul, 2016.

11. "H724 - 'aruwkah - Strong's Hebrew Lexicon (KJV)."
    Blue Letter Bible. Web. 15 Jul, 2016.

12. "G2323 - therapeuō - Strong's Greek Lexicon (KJV)."
    Blue Letter Bible. Web. 13 Jul, 2016.

13. "G2390 - iaomai - Strong's Greek Lexicon (KJV)." Blue
    Letter Bible. Web. 13 Jul, 2016.

14. "G2386 - iama - Strong's Greek Lexicon (KJV)." Blue
    Letter Bible. Web. 13 Jul, 2016.

15. "G2392 - iasis - Strong's Greek Lexicon (KJV)." Blue
    Letter Bible. Web. 13 Jul, 2016.

16. "G4982 - sōzō - Strong's Greek Lexicon (KJV)." Blue
    Letter Bible. Web. 13 Jul, 2016.

17. "G1295 - diasōzō - Strong's Greek Lexicon (KJV)." Blue
    Letter Bible. Web. 13 Jul, 2016.

18. "G5198 - hygiainō - Strong's Greek Lexicon (KJV)."

Blue Letter Bible. Web. 15 Jul, 2016.

Appendix Three

1. "H7822 - shĕchiyn - Strong's Hebrew Lexicon (KJV)." Blue Letter Bible. Web. 6 Sep, 2016.

2. "G1420 - dysenteria - Strong's Greek Lexicon (KJV)." Blue Letter Bible. Web. 6 Sep, 2016.

3. "H7829 - shachepheth - Strong's Hebrew Lexicon (KJV)." Blue Letter Bible. Web. 6 Sep, 2016.

4. "artho-". *Dictionary.com Unabridged.* Random House, Inc. 6 Sep. 2016.

5. "-itis". *Dictionary.com Unabridged.* Random House, Inc. 6 Sep. 2016.

6. "BibleGateway." *Deut 28:65 NIV.* N.p., n.d. Web. 06 Sept. 2016.

7. "BibleGateway." *Deut 28:65 CEB.* N.p., n.d. Web. 06 Sept. 2016.

8. "H1816 - dalleqeth - Strong's Hebrew Lexicon (KJV)." Blue Letter Bible. Web. 6 Sep, 2016.

9. "H2914 - tĕchor - Strong's Hebrew Lexicon (KJV)." Blue Letter Bible. Web. 6 Sep, 2016.

10. Online, Catholic Bible. "Knox Bible." Knox Bible. N.p., n.d. Web. 06 Sept. 2016.

11. "H1698 - deber - Strong's Hebrew Lexicon (KJV)." Blue Letter Bible. Web. 6 Sep, 2016.

12. "H3420 - yeraqown - Strong's Hebrew Lexicon (KJV)." Blue Letter Bible. Web. 6 Sep, 2016.

13. "H6920 - qaddachath - Strong's Hebrew Lexicon (KJV)." Blue Letter Bible. Web. 6 Sep, 2016.

14. "H8270 - shor - Strong's Hebrew Lexicon (KJV)." Blue Letter Bible. Web. 6 Sep, 2016.

15. "H990 - beten - Strong's Hebrew Lexicon (KJV)." Blue Letter Bible. Web. 6 Sep, 2016.

16. "H1618 - garab - Strong's Hebrew Lexicon (KJV)." Blue Letter Bible. Web. 6 Sep, 2016.

17. "H2775 - cherec - Strong's Hebrew Lexicon (KJV)." Blue Letter Bible. Web. 6 Sep, 2016.

18. "H2746 - charchur - Strong's Hebrew Lexicon (KJV)." Blue Letter Bible. Web. 6 Sep, 2016.

ABOUT THE AUTHOR

TIMOTHY J. SABO is a former graduate of Rhema Bible Training College in Tulsa, Oklahoma. Author, missionary, and Spirit-filled preacher of the Word, Timothy currently teaches wherever he goes, bringing in piles of Word of Faith materials and building lending libraries in churches, Bible colleges and wherever the door opens around the world.

Timothy and Jaime Sabo reside in Canada with their two daughters.